QUICKIES

ONE HUNDRED LITTLE LESSONS FOR LIVING SEXILY EVER AFTER IN MIDLIFE

HEATHER BARTOS, MD

Empress Editions N° 1
Published by Empress Editions LLC 2025
First Printing

copyright © 2025 Heather Bartos, MD
All rights reserved.

Typeset in Baskerville in Cambridge.
Printed and bound in New York by Vicks.

ISBN 979-8-992386-509

Empress Editions
303 Third Street
Cambridge, MA 02142
+1 617.580.5266

www.empresseditions.net

Endpapers taken from the exquisite design *Bosque Dreams* by Emma J Shipley. Inspired by Emma's travels in the Osa Peninsula in Costa Rica, one of the most biodiverse places on Earth. An enigmatic puma stands centre-stage, surrounded by other fantastical creatures of the forest, including macaws, monkeys, sloths, ocelots and more. Other influences include Pre-Raphaelite paintings, mid-19th century Arts and Crafts movement textiles, and Edward Lear illustrations.

Reproduced with kind permission of the artist.
Our sincerest thanks to her.

www.emmajshipley.com

© Emma J Shipley Ltd 2025

Since it would be wildly inappropriate to dedicate a book about midlife sex to my amazing, supportive family (love you!) . . .

To the gals who were told their bodies were too much or not enough, who were made to believe desire fades with time, or that their best years were behind them—

To the women who've ever felt invisible, who were told their pleasure was secondary, and who've spent too much time apologizing for the space they take up in this world—

To the ladies who have felt unseen, unheard, and unvalidated—like their desires, their voices, and their worth were somehow negotiable—

I dedicate this book to you, love. I see you.

"I sing the body electric. . ."
    —Walt Whitman and *Fame*, because pleasure, passion, and power deserve a damn good soundtrack.

FOREWORD

BY YOUR VAGINA

Oh hey there. It's me—your vagina.

I know, I know. You weren't expecting to hear from me in the foreword of a book, were you? But here I am, front and center (for once), ready to say what we've both been thinking: It's about time.

Listen, we've been through a lot together. Remember the good ol' times? The spontaneous nights, the steamy mornings, the occasional (okay, frequent) skinny dips and risky business in public places? Yeah, those were the days. But then life happened—jobs, kids, midlife crises, hot flashes (and not the fun kind). Suddenly, I became less of a star and more of a... supporting character.

But darling, let me be clear: I'm still here. And trust me, I've got more to give.

That's why this book, *Quickies: 100 Little Lessons for Living Sexily Ever After in Midlife*, is your new best friend. It's not just about sex (though, trust me, we're into that). It's about rediscovering pleasure—in every sense of the word. It's about savoring life's little thrills, reigniting the spark, and realizing that midlife isn't the end of the road—it's the start of a whole new adventure.

And let's be honest, I've been a bit neglected lately. Sure, I'm resilient, but a little attention never hurt anyone. This book is your permission slip to flirt with life again—to embrace the quickies, the slow burns, and everything in between.

So go on, turn the page. Let's get reacquainted.

Love always,
Your Vagina

QUICK & DIRTY

YOUR GUIDE TO GETTING THE MOST OUT OF THIS BOOK

Hello midlife mavens!

Welcome to the 'sexily ever after' book of *you*. For far too long, we've been the 'good girls,' bending ourselves into shapes that please everyone *but* ourselves. That needs to stop! It's time to hit pause on that performative bull crap. Instead, grab a mock-tail (or whatever makes you feel deliciously alive) and indulge in *Quickies*.

What is *Quickies*, you politely ask?

Sister, THIS is your private midlife playbook of the divine feminine, stashed away in the secret drawer of your inner world. For your eyes—and your hands (and all of your senses) —only. *Quickies* is where you get to explore, feel, and voice your truth with zero apologies or filters. In this sacred space, you can finally strip off every mask and stand fully in the glow of your unvarnished self. YOUR truth. Remember the maxim: authentic intimacy isn't about taking off your clothes, it's about taking off your "I'm fine." That hits hard, am I right? It's being naked in ways that maybe have nothing to do with skin, but are more alluring than ever. Yowza. Deep breath, loves.

To this end, *Quickies* is divided into three illuminating sections. These 'shorts' all derive from the award-winning and über-popular podcast *The SEX Podcast* by yours truly. With more than 200 episodes over three years of helping women find their own intimate voice . . . the culmination of those stories now lies in your hot little hands. This book came into existence because we knew there were so many women to reach, and more than ONE BILLION of us are in midlife.

The first section tackles the *un*learning—shedding all the outdated, patriarchal myths about pleasure, intimacy, and sexual satisfaction that traditional sex ed tried to drill into us. The second dives into *sexploration*, offering playful and practical insights on how to embrace your kinks and curiosities without a trace of shame. In fact, zero shame can be found in this book; I can't stand that word! And the third and final section delivers straight-from-the-expert wisdom, where this board-certified gynecologist breaks down the taboos and hush-hush topics no one wants to discuss—until we make them not only discussable but downright empowering with facts, revolutionary compassion, and a healthy dose of no-nonsense advice. Tough talk from your rah-rah bestie here, because let's face it: everybody's got *something* at some point.

Think of this book as a provocative thought experiment in radical self-acceptance. A *Vanity Fair*-style profile with you as both the probing journalist and the fascinating subject (and fantastic cover shoot in some glorious outfit of your choosing). Some moments will feel delightfully serendipitous, like spotting constellations in spilled tea leaves. Others are carefully crafted to tease out truths you've yet to notice about yourself.

It's a game, a sexily-ever-after journey—starring you. The only rule, my sister? Complete. Radical. Honesty.

No one's watching but you, so how brave can you be? How loud can you sing? How hard can you dance (I know you are amazing at all of these, because I believe in the visionary power of women!)

Before you dive in, slow your roll for just a sec. Imagine you're standing on the edge of a cliff, ready to leap into uncharted waters (without sharks, because I can't even). Consider these sacred precepts of our *Quickies* collective:

- I will explore the labyrinth of my mind and body, unlocking the doors to my pleasure.
- I will fiercely and unapologetically speak my truth when it comes to my desires.
- I will embrace the life-altering magic of "'not giving a f**k'" but definitely giving a *flick* through this book to guide me on this journey of sexual self-discovery.

If you're ready to honor these audacious and freeing principles, congratulations—you're one of us: bold, beautiful, and utterly unflinching midlife goddesses. And I knew you were.

Proclaim allegiance to your fully realized, fully sensual self.

Now, just turn the page. Or let the majestic universe turn it for you. And as Annie Lennox and Aretha Franklin so wisely sang, tell yourself: "Sisters are doing it for themselves."

PART I
THE UNLEARNING

Shedding outdated, patriarchal myths about pleasure, intimacy, and sexual satisfaction.

LESSON ONE

SEXY AF AT ANY AGE: WHY MIDLIFE IS AN EPIC MILESTONE

RIGHT HERE, right now, it's time to have an important revelation: midlife is an evolution. Yes, retiree organizations like AARP may start sending you magazines, and yes, the world will offer you discounts on senior coffees at fast food joints. Screw that! (But I'll take the free cup of Joe.) This chapter is a celebration of how turning fifty—and every year after—is an opportunity to unlock a deeper, richer version of sexy. If you're reading this in advance of fifty (say, forty, forty-five, or even thirty-eight)—congrats to you, because you're not going down lightly. I do love a woman of action!!

Let's start with inspiration. Take a moment to think of some well-known women we admire: Angela Bassett, Sandra Bullock, Michelle Yeoh, and Helen Mirren, just to name a few. What do these women have in common? Yes, they are objectively gorgeous. But more importantly, they embody agency (and they are also getting propaganda for 'active senior communities'). They take charge of their lives, unapologetically own their stories, and nurture a deep connection with themselves. Some have had their best careers post-fifty. Their visibility reminds us that sexy isn't confined to a number—it's a mindset, a commitment to self-respect, and an embrace of life's ever-evolving journey.

What's the secret sauce to staying sexy in your fifties, sixties, and beyond? It's not about trying to defy gravity (although a little help never hurts), it's about leaning into what makes you feel alive and radiant. For some, that might mean skincare rituals or hormone therapy. For others, it's finding joy in the little glimmers of daily life—like a great pair of shoes, a bold lipstick, or even a well-earned laugh about gravity's effect on certain body parts. Some women are emboldened by their wisdom, the gray hair, and the smile lines.

And let's talk about self-care, or as I like to call it "self-respect"—because nothing says sexy like owning your health. When I had my first colonoscopy, while the prep was an adventure (hello, Beyonce-inspired detox!), I walked out of that clinic feeling empowered. Groggy, but empowered! Taking care of yourself—mind, body, and soul—isn't just responsible; it's downright attractive.

But sexy isn't just about how you look or what you do. It's about the stories you carry and the wisdom you share. As women, we have a collective wealth of experiences—decades of love, loss, triumph, and transformation. Sharing those stories, those 'sexy glimmers,' with each other and with younger generations creates a ripple effect. We pass down confidence, knowledge, and the audacity to live fully at every age.

So, here's the challenge: find what makes *you* feel sexy, and own it. Look away from the nubile twenty-year-old influencers. Find yours, whether it's a daily ritual, a fearless outfit, or simply deciding not to give a damn about things that don't serve you anymore. Share your secrets, your wisdom, and your 'aha' moments because together, we're shaping the narrative of what it means to be a sexy, powerful woman at fifty and beyond.

Remember, sexy has never been about perfection. It's about connection—being deeply attuned to yourself and unapologetically authentic. And if we can show the next generation how it's done, we're not just aging gracefully—we're aging *sexfully*.

LESSON TWO

SHOULD YOU QUIT SEX FOR GOOD?
(SPOILER: HELL NO.)

So, here's an interesting question: should you quit sex for good? Don't panic, sister!

Let me reframe the question.

Does sex, as it's currently showing up in your life, serve you—mind, body, and spirit? (Put another way, are you planning your Walmart shopping list while doin' the deed? Oh wait, we need glue sticks, butter, and more laundry detergent . . . sound familiar?)

Does it align with your desires, your truths, and your evolving identity? Maybe you no longer want to tolerate bad oral. Or scratchy stubble. Or boring lube choices.

Or has it become something you endure; a relic of expectations you no longer share? (*To be a 'good partner' I should just give it up and put up with it. I'll just lay here because that makes me compliant.* Ummm, no, but that's another lesson for another day.)

The question of QUIET QUITTING on sex is all around us, like South Korea's 4B movement—which advocates for women to reject relationships and procreation with dudes—to celibate celebrities like Jane Fonda, Diane Keaton, Julia Fox,

Mariah Carey, and even Lady Gaga. (Now, they haven't called to tell me about their sex retirement, but it's all over Google if you believe everything you read.) Even Drew Barrymore has laid it open about not getting laid.

So let's say, "We're on a break."

Okay, for how long? The phrase "for good" is layered. Is it forever? Or is it for the better? In *Wicked*, when Glinda and Elphaba sing of being changed "for good," it has a dual meaning—a permanent transformation and an improvement. And then we fly off on a magnificent broom and change Oz. Oh, wait. Wrong story.

So when we consider giving up sex, let's hold space for both interpretations. Could you–could any of us–let go of sex forever? Most of us didn't sign up for that, à la Mother Teresa. Or would stepping away for now lead you to a better place— emotionally, spiritually, and even physically?

THE EVOLVING MEANING OF SEX

Sex used to seem like such an easy concept. But as we age (gorgeously, of course), we are apt to bend the notion of what sex can be for us. Take octogenarian Jane Fonda. After three marriages, she has declared that she loves being by herself and no longer desires sexual relationships. With the wrong partner, sex is boring and a waste of time . . . and midlife women value their time more than anything. We know our finiteness, and if we can't have the whole crème brûlée, we'd rather not take a bite of Jello. But hey . . . if Jane meets a much younger man? She says she'd be open to playing the field again (and presumably aiming for a Grand Slam), but she'd want to play with a younger team. MEANING: IF she decides to have sex again, it won't be an obligation, it will be for pleasure and joy on her terms.

And what about you? What do you really want from sex?

It's no longer a quick romp in the back of a Trans Am listening to Bon Jovi. We've been improving, maturing, and growing and we want ... MORE.

What do you truly want from sex? There's a point where nearly every woman I see takes a massive PAUSE on sex (I personally think Mother Nature provides this for us so we can take an accounting of what the heck we want now that procreation is off the table). And in that pause, we began to assess: What serves me now? What feels authentic? What brings me pleasure, connection, and meaning?

A good friend of mine who is a sex therapist always asks women how they would take their perfect cup of coffee (or tea). What's the temperature? Is it Espresso? Americano? Are you a coconut or oat milk gal? Lavender or hazelnut syrup maybe? Or sugar in the raw. Only when you can describe your perfect cup of joe can you then proceed to have a perfect cup of Joe/Jo. (See what I did there?)

A NEW DEFINITION OF PLEASURE

Stepping away from sex *with a partner* doesn't mean abandoning pleasure. Heck to the no. It means redefining it. It means reclaiming your agency and rewriting your narrative. There's nothing sexier than a woman who knows herself. So let's do it:

- Is sex as I know it adding to my life?
- Am I craving emotional intimacy, physical connection, or both?
- What does pleasure mean to me—and how can I cultivate it on my terms?
- Has anyone ever asked you this before? Because no one had asked me, that's for dang sure.

We won't settle for less, but rather raise the bar. At midlife, we value quality over quantity. Let's face it, ~~many~~ most women find that the pool of potential partners feels lackluster or mismatched with the depth of our inner growth. You don't pair a fine wine with a red Solo cup. We're not judging! It's clarity. If the people you're meeting aren't coming to the table with authenticity, generosity, and emotional availability, it's okay to step back.

LIVING SEXY WITHOUT SEX

Let me also just bring it into the audience for a moment: saying no to sex doesn't mean saying no to being sexy. You can still feel vibrant, alive, and magnetic without a partner or traditional notions of physical intimacy.

Instead, you might focus on:

- **Inner sexy:** Developing a deep connection with yourself—your body, your desires, and your essence. This book is a great start.
- **Soulful pleasure:** What lights you up from the inside? What colors your world with joy? Did all of us think that books like *Fifty Shades* fell flat for what we desire most?
- **Self-love rituals:** Indulge in self-pleasure, pamper your body, or try practices like meditation, dance, or tantra. Any dance that moves those hips (think Samba, Bollywood, belly dancing) opens up the blood flow to that area.

QUITTING SEX . . . INTENTIONALLY

If you're going to quit sex, do it with intention. Like a great movie, the heroine tells the entire board of directors to "F off" in the most dramatic fashion and then walks out of the ground floor glass doors, spins around, and throws up her hat Mary Tyler Moore-style. Think of the finale of *Working Girl*,

Devil Wears Prada, and Legally Blonde. At least, that's how I think of it.

Ask yourself:

- Am I stepping back to date and fall in love with myself?
- Am I clearing out old narratives and Marie Kondo-ing my emotional closet? We will work on this!
- Am I exploring new realms of pleasure, connection, and fulfillment?

For each reason, identify what you're gaining in return. Assign a color, a flavor, a sensation. What word embodies this new chapter? Is it freedom? Radiance? Serenity?

THE FINAL QUESTION

Yes, you can give up sex. But what do you plan to give yourself in its place? Whether it's spiritual fulfillment, radical self-love, lack of pregnancy or STI, or simply peace, let your decision come from a place of empowerment, not deprivation. Let it reflect what's 'for good'—for the better, for the now, for the you that you're becoming.

Now, I'm craving a cup of coffee.

LESSON THREE

WHY YOU DON'T FEEL SEXY—AND HOW TO FIX IT

Time for a radical truth.

Sexy is not a size, a number on a scale, or a perfect photo-op pose. (bent leg in front, tuck that arm flab back, chins UP! Don't forget to breathe.)

It's not a crazy high libido or wrinkle-free skin. Thinking otherwise is as absurd as saying you don't have a real relationship unless you never fight or you're not a parent unless your children behave impeccably.

Say it with me: *You can be over forty-five and still be sexy.* You can have back pain, extra pounds, stretch marks, or even a rash and still be sexy. Sexy is not about fitting into someone else's definition—it's about creating your own.

THE PROBLEM: A CULTURE OF PERFECTION

Our struggle with sexiness begins with a cultural myth that equates beauty with flawlessness. This myth is everywhere: in ads, media, and childhood whispers. For decades, women have been sold the idea that sexy looks like Marilyn Monroe in the '50s, Twiggy in the '60s, or the heroin chic of Kate Moss in the '90s. Today, it might be a 700-calorie-a-day celebrity-inspired 'cleanse.' But these ideals come with a hidden cost: eating disorders, low self-esteem, and emotional exhaustion.

For generations, women who seemed sexy on the outside —from Judy Garland to Princess Diana—suffered silently behind the scenes. Their struggles reveal a stark truth: the gap between *looking sexy* and *feeling sexy* is vast.

And yet, many of us internalize these impossible standards, believing we're not enough. A global study by Dove revealed that 70 percent of women feel that media and advertising set unrealistic expectations of beauty. Worse, this belief starts young: self-esteem in girls peaks at age nine. NINE. After that, the toxic cultural narrative chips away at confidence, leaving women to grapple with self-doubt that impacts their education, careers, and relationships.

THE SOLUTION: REDEFINE SEXY FOR YOURSELF

Here's the good news: you don't have to stay stuck in this cycle. The antidote to the culture's toxic definition of sexy is simple but profound—you must define sexy *for yourself.*

This means shedding outdated ideas and creating space for a version of sexy that aligns with who you are. Doing so isn't just about feeling better in your skin; it's a revolution that uplifts your daughters, nieces, and every woman who sees you boldly embracing yourself.

START WITH THESE TWO STEPS:

CELEBRATE WHAT YOU LOVE ABOUT YOURSELF

Sexy starts with self-acceptance. It's not about changing yourself to fit a mold but finding joy in what makes you uniquely you. Remember that little girl who loved sparkly shoes? She still lives inside you. Nurture her curiosity, her courage, and her flair for the fabulous.

FIND ROLE MODELS OF REAL SEXY

Make a list of ten women you find sexy—women who embody confidence, authenticity, and vitality. They can be celebrities, activists, neighbors, or friends. Maybe it's Betty White's randy hilariousness at any age, Serena Williams's unapologetic power, or Rita Moreno's fire. Ask yourself: *What makes them magnetic to me?* Write it down. This is a great game to play with a set of girlfriends, which contains zero calories.

By admiring these women's specific traits, you're rewiring your brain. This practice, called neuroplasticity, teaches you to see beauty beyond the superficial, paving the way to recognize it in yourself.

SEXY IS A STATE OF MIND

Sexy isn't about age, weight, or a blowout hairstyle. Sexy is Eleanor Roosevelt owning her brilliance. It's Angela Lansbury radiating confidence at ninety-three. It's you, stepping into your power.

So start today. Look in the mirror and remind yourself:

- Sexy isn't a size; it's a spirit.
- Sexy isn't extra credit; it's a daily birthright.
- Sexy is as sexy does.

And remember, when you stop looking for sexy *out there* and start nurturing it within, you won't just see it in yourself—you'll find it everywhere.

LESSON FOUR

SEX VALUES: YOUR SECRET WEAPON FOR UNSTOPPABLE SEXY

To LIVE SEXILY EVER after in midlife, we must begin with a fundamental truth: clarity about our sexual values is the foundation of fulfilling an authentic sexual identity. Our values—whether about life or sexuality—guide our choices, illuminate our priorities, and reveal the essence of what matters most to us. But how often have we paused to consider our *sexual* values? Probably not often enough, and I certainly don't recommend doing it while organizing your closet, unless you don't really want to organize said closet.

WHY VALUES MATTER

Values are not mere words; they're the compass that guides us through tough decisions and helps us navigate conflicts between desire and reality. When it comes to sexuality, knowing our values makes it easier to set boundaries, articulate desires, and create meaningful connections. Without this clarity, we risk acting outside of our comfort zones, often leading to shame, guilt, or regret. And this opens us up to relationships with narcissists, sociopaths, and other negative entities.

But hold the phone: most of us never had a proper sexual

education. I mean, have you ever put a condom on a banana *since* high school? Our early lessons about sex—whether from parents, peers, or media—were often laced with awkwardness, misinformation, or silence. I always thought *Schoolhouse Rock* missed a tremendous opportunity to train our generation about sex, because I knew way more about 'conjunction junction' then 'erection connection.' I am proud to report I know how a bill gets into law, though. Understanding our sexual values can help undo this legacy of discomfort and replace it with a sense of ownership and pride.

THE SPECTRUM OF SEXUAL VALUES

Once, a fascinating study of college students identified three broad sexual value systems: absolutism (abstinence until marriage), relativism (sexual decisions based on relationships), and hedonism (if it feels good, do it). The researchers looked at age of the student, ethnicity, etc. But only three? The most common value that was selected? Relativism (Always choose door number two). Because it's the middle of the road, where most people could accept it.

But we're way past college-aged studies! As midlife women, we can do better. Let's consider values like trust, kindness, creativity, humor, and authenticity—universal principles that can be applied to our sexual selves.

For instance, I discovered that some of my general life values—creativity and kindness—also resonated with my sexual identity. However, I also identified new values, like trust and collaboration, that were uniquely tied to my intimate life. This exercise was transformative, revealing how deeply our sexual values intertwine with our overall sense of self. I even found that financial responsibility was tied to my intimate life, because if I felt more secure in my everyday life, I was more likely to feel open and vulnerable in le boudoir.

HOW TO IDENTIFY YOUR SEXUAL VALUES

Okay, so enough about me. Are you ready to find yours? Start here:

1. What makes me feel sexually confident and fulfilled?
2. What turns me on? What satisfies me sexually?
3. What are my boundaries? Where do I draw the line?
4. How do I define a positive sexual experience?

Oh, and for the record, you don't have to write these out. You can jam out on your phone, computer, voice notes, whatever works for you. Now we create. Think of words that *resonate with you*: integrity, playfulness, generosity, self-respect, peace, curiosity. Don't overthink it; choose six to eight core values that feel authentic and meaningful. This list is not set in stone, so you can amend or revise it to your heart's content.

SHARING YOUR VALUES

If you have a partner, sharing your sexual values can be a game-changer. You'll want to call it foreplay if they're a guy. Think of it as offering them a roadmap to your pleasure and intimacy. For example, if collaboration is a core value, your partner might recognize the importance of shared effort in initiating and enjoying intimacy. This process deepens connection and makes navigating differences easier. No, truly, once they share theirs, they'll see the magic that comes (?) from knowing each other's. And if you don't have a partner, GREAT! You'll walk into a future relationship knowing exactly your taste of tea. Display them where you'll see them daily, or revisit them regularly to remind yourself of your authentic sexual identity. Over time, these values will become an integral part of how you move through the world—not just in the bedroom but in your entire life.

VALUES IN ACTION

Like cleaning a closet, identifying your sexual values is not a one and done task. They're not static; they WILL evolve as you grow and change. What feels important today might shift in a year or a decade, with a new relationship or hormonal change. Embrace this evolution with curiosity. Your values are not just about sex but about how you feel sexy—a state of being that transcends the act itself. Whew, that sounded super deep.

Living sexily ever after in midlife starts with understanding YOU. Because who taught us how to do that? When you're clear about your sexual values, you give yourself permission to be authentic, confident, and unapologetically you. And that's the secret to a life filled with connection, joy, and lasting intimacy.

LESSON FIVE

THOU SHALT HONOR THY CELLULITE, FAT, AND FUPA

Ah, cellulite, fat, and the FUPA (the 'fat upper pubic area' or, if you prefer, the 'fat upper pussy area'). Once whispered about in shame, now brought into the light by none other than Queen Beyoncé, who famously embraced her "mommy pouch" in a 2018 *Vogue* essay. If a pop superstar can name it, claim it, and love it, why shouldn't we? Let's zip down the low-rise jeans on this trifecta of midlife intimacy saboteurs—and learn to honor them instead.

RECLAIM THE NARRATIVE: THE BEAUTY OF CELLULITE

Did you know that up to 98 percent of women have cellulite? The other 2 percent were probably lost on the way to the research study. To sum it up: that's nearly all of us, ladies. Those dimples are not a flaw; they're a feature—a reflection of the unique architecture of female bodies. French women, often lauded for their effortless allure, have a word for it too: la peau d'orange (orange peel skin). I mean, even the French acknowledge that it's as common as croissants.

So, what if instead of fighting cellulite, we embraced it? After all, dimples on your cheeks are charming, so why not consider your legs and thighs as equally endearing? Skip the overpriced creams. If you want to dry-brush or massage with coconut oil, do it because it feels sensual—not because you're trying to erase something Mother Nature gave the female form.

FAT IS NOT THE ENEMY

Fat has become the worst of the 'F-words,' a source of endless guilt and shame, yet it's also part of the natural ebb and flow of life. Historically, fuller bodies were considered signs of fertility, abundance, and desirability. Even today, preferences vary: search for "BBW" (Big Beautiful Women) online, and you'll find an entire category celebrating voluptuousness. Flemish Painter Paul Rubens preferred to paint his epic heroines with round waists, and curvy hips, and breasts. Thus, the term "Rubensesque" was born to describe this body type.

Your partner likely finds your curves far more inviting than you think. And if you're struggling to feel sexy, remember: confidence is the real aphrodisiac. A black lace bra and an oversized button-down crisp white shirt (strategically unbuttoned) can work wonders. So can dim lighting, flattering positions, and a playful attitude.

FUPA: FROM TABOO TO TROPHY

The pop star's celebration of her FUPA helped to reframe this little-understood feature of the female form. Whether it's a result of childbirth, genetics, or a love of pasta, the FUPA is not your enemy. As Fabienne in *Pulp Fiction* so eloquently put it, "I would actually wear a t-shirt two sizes too small to accentuate it."

That confidence? That's what's sexy.

If low-rise jeans make you shudder, opt for high-waisted elegance instead. If a FUPA feels like a stumbling block during intimacy, try waist-slimming positions like doggy style or simply focus on the sensations rather than the aesthetics. Your partner's gaze isn't critiquing; it's adoring.

THREE TIPS FOR FEELING LESS SELF-CONSCIOUS ABOUT YOUR BODY DURING INTIMACY

1. **Shift the Spotlight**: Stop magnifying your insecurities. Instead, focus on the pleasure of touch, connection, and shared desire. When your mind is fully present, self-consciousness fades.
2. **Dress for Desire**: Find lingerie or outfits that make you feel confident. A plunging neckline, soft satin robe, or even a playful costume can transform your mindset and keep you engaged in the moment.
3. **Create a Mood**: Soft lighting, sensual scents, and music can help you relax and get out of your head. Dim the lights, put on a playlist that makes you feel like a goddess, and let go of the inner critic.

Your body isn't the villain in your love story—it's the main attraction. Every curve, dimple, and jiggle is part of the masterpiece that makes you *you*. That soft belly? A VIP lounge for pleasure. Those thighs? Thunderous applause for a life well lived. Stop fighting the very thing that delivers the magic —celebrate it, flaunt it, and let it lead you to the good stuff.

LESSON SIX

SAYING GOODBYE TO SELF-BLAME IN THE BEDROOM

IMAGINE yourself standing in front of a mirror, owning every angle of your reflection. Not with blame, not with excuses, but with clear-eyed accountability. This is where we begin: shedding the victim card and rewriting the script of your inner sexy monologue.

WHY BANISHING BLAME IS SEXY

I get it. Victimhood may feel comforting at first. It's easy to point fingers; to wallow in the 'why me' of it all. But this mindset steals your power, saps your sex appeal, and chains you to inaction. It's a mindset many of us were taught growing up: the damsel in distress. Owning your narrative, however, is electrifying. It's the spark that lights the fire of self-confidence, resilience, and yes, even desire. The question isn't, "Can I stop playing the victim?" but rather, "Am I ready to reclaim my life?"

THREE STEPS TO DITCH THE VICTIM COMPLEX AND
EMBRACE OWNERSHIP

1. **Ask Yourself: What Do I Really Want?** Every change begins with clarity. Define your goals. What is it you truly want? Maybe it's rekindling intimacy with your partner, embracing a healthier lifestyle, or simply feeling in control of your body and mind. Make it concrete: "I want to connect with my partner one night a week" is a tangible goal you can work toward. Abstract wishes like "I want to feel better" will only keep you stuck.

2. **Transform Your Internal Dialogue**. That inner voice? It needs a makeover. Instead of spiraling into self-pity or frustration, call out your complaints playfully. Try a dramatic accent or exaggerate them until they're laughable. This reframing transforms a tantrum into a moment of levity and perspective. Replace defeatist thoughts (*I'll never feel sexy again*) with realistic truths (*I'm learning to prioritize my desires*). The shift from victimhood to empowerment is subtle but seismic.

3. **Take Small, Intentional Actions**. Ownership is built one small victory at a time. Start with manageable steps: make a list of priorities, educate yourself on your health, or schedule a fun, flirty date with yourself or your partner. Whether it's learning how your body works post-menopause or finding a dance routine (yes!) that excites you, these actions chip away at shame and build confidence. Remember, the key isn't perfection but persistence.

LIVING THE REWRITE: FROM EXCUSES TO EMPOWERMENT

When you catch yourself falling into old patterns of blame, pause. Take stock of the situation and rewrite the story. Did your lab results not improve this quarter? Rather than listing excuses ("It was my sister's wedding"), acknowledge your choices: "I indulged a bit, but I see where I can make adjustments moving forward." This isn't about perfection; it's about progress.

Empowerment doesn't mean you'll never slip. Hell, no! That's a load of crap if someone promises you that. Some days, you'll find yourself knee-deep in the manure of self-pity. That's okay. What matters is shaking off the crusted poo, getting back on the horse, and riding forward. It's resilience that makes the difference—not the absence of failure but the refusal to let it define you.

NEW TOOLS FOR A NEW NARRATIVE

Empowered living means identifying the tools and resources you need. Maybe it's a community with like-oriented goals, a coach, or even a beautifully organized checklist on a quirky notepad of kittens holding colored pencils. What works for someone else might not work for you, and that's okay. The key is to find what aligns with your unique rhythm and goals.

As you fill your life with proactive energy, you'll notice something remarkable: the space once occupied by blame and shame is now fertile ground for growth, connection, and yes, a more vibrant, sexy you. Which is exactly what we're aiming for here!

CLOSING THOUGHTS: OWN IT, SISTER

What you focus on expands. If you're mired in blame and shame, you'll attract more of the same. But if you're intentional about growth, accountability, and joy, you'll see those qualities flourish. Every challenge is an opportunity to rewrite your story. Every moment is a chance to reclaim your power. So, let's amputate that victim card and step boldly into a life of confidence and connection.

Your new mantra: *I own my life. I own my choices. I own my sexy. And I deserve all the beauty and pleasure this world has to offer.*

LESSON SEVEN

THE DRY SPELL: HOW TO REKINDLE (OR RELEASE) A SEXLESS PARTNERSHIP

THE SEXLESS RELATIONSHIP. Something we don't discuss often enough. We're talking *no* intimacy. Nada. None. Not the kind where you're both contentedly coasting on companionship, but the kind where one of you is playing "Sweet Dreams" on repeat while the other is lying awake, wondering if this is how we die.

You've pulled out all the stops. A spritz of your go-to seduction perfume, a slinky silk nightgown that hasn't seen the light of day in a decade, and a wax that nearly had you calling for an epidural. I even one time let them wax the 'honey pot,' which is the butt if you're interested in knowing. There, now we're best friends. You've hinted at romantic getaways, maybe even suggested a little afternoon delight—but all you get is a polite kiss ON THE CHEEK, a "Goodnight, dear," and the cold shoulder. And then snoring. SNORING. How rude.

Here's the thing: we've been conditioned to believe that our partners are always ready and raring to go. So when they aren't, we assume the problem is . . . us. We spiral into self-doubt. Am I too old? Too fat? Too unfuckable? Spoiler alert: It's not you, babe. It's them.

WHEN DESIRE DRIES UP: THE "MANOPAUSE" MYSTERY

Now this section is for my gals who are in relationships with men—welcome to the world of andropause (or as I like to call it, "*man*opause"). Just like us, men experience hormonal changes, stress, and life upheavals that can tank their libido. But I feel sorry for the dudes—HEAR ME OUT! Unlike us, they don't have a culture of support or an arsenal of self-help books to guide them. They rarely even go to the doctor unless their partner has scheduled it (and even then it's like dragging a toddler to shot day). Instead, they're left with a dwindling desire and no language to express it. Poor guys.

And let's not forget the emotional baggage. Maybe your partner is grappling with unresolved shame, body image issues, a past history of abuse (it's way more common than we'd like to admit), or stress from work. But if we're honest, knowing the 'why' doesn't make rejection any easier. It feels so damn personal. Painfully so. All those tropes about 'them always wanting it' make us feel utterly alone. And frankly, unsexy.

THE TRUTH ABOUT INTIMACY (AND WHY IT'S NOT JUST ABOUT SEX)

A sexless relationship isn't just about the lack of sex; it's about the absence of intimacy—the gentle touches, stolen glances, and whispered confessions that make us feel cherished. When those go missing, resentment creeps in, and she's a bitch. We start to actually believe that we're unworthy, unlovable, or invisible. We love to feel . . . wanted.

I've been there. For nearly two years, my marriage was a desert, and I was parched. Here's the breakdown: I blamed myself, then blamed him, him some more, then more of him, and cycled right back to blaming myself. Are you dizzy yet? It took a toll on my confidence, my relationships, and my sense of self. But here's the good news: there's a way through this. You don't have to stay stuck in the dry spell.

THREE TIPS FOR SURVIVING (AND THRIVING) IN A SEXLESS RELATIONSHIP

1. **Reclaim Your Sexy—for You**. Stop waiting for external validation. I know a lot of us are guilty of the ol' "how do I look?" and when they grunt approval or don't even look up from their phone, it's utter disappointment. But sister, darling lady . . . your desirability doesn't hinge on someone else's libido. Invest in whatever makes *you* feel alive and radiant. Dance in your underwear. Buy the lingerie, even if no one else sees it. Once I stopped asking how I looked, it's amazing how fast the compliments started coming. Walk out of the closet and say, "Damn, I look fine." Own your sexy because it's yours—not theirs.

2. **Have the Hard (oooh bad pun) Conversation**. Yes, it's awkward. But nothing changes if you don't talk. Approach your partner with curiosity, not criticism. Instead of, "Why don't you want me anymore?" try, "I've noticed we haven't been connecting physically. Can we explore why?" Vulnerability opens doors; blame slams them shut. Learn from me: chasing them to various rooms of the house looking for answers doesn't get you answers.

3. **Seek Support Together.** My two favorite books that I read at this time were: *It Takes One to Tango* by Marriage Therapist Winifred M. Reilly, who suffered her own humiliating relationship issue. *Extreme Ownership* by former Navy Seals Jocko Willink and Leif Babbitt. Betcha never thought

you'd see those together in a book on female sexuality (pretty sure they didn't either)! I'm gonna say it outright: Screw couples' counseling. Not permanently, but going every week and picking off a scab doesn't make a wound heal faster. It just makes you bleed and more prone to infection. Fix yourself first. Only then do you have the strength and resilience to help the group (it's like putting your oxygen mask on first).

YOUR INNER KOMODO DRAGON AWAITS

A sexless marriage can feel like a betrayal of the connection you once had. But it's also an opportunity. It's a chance to confront the myths we've internalized about desire, intimacy, and self-worth. Let's look at an unlikely avatar for ourselves: the Komodo dragon. She hates dealing with partner drama so much she can get sexual without one. So can you.

So, sister, if you're lying there wondering whether this is your life for the next fifty years, let me tell you: it doesn't have to be. Whether you rekindle the flame, find peace in the companionship, or choose a different path a la Komodo, the most important thing is this—you deserve to feel cherished, desired, and deeply connected. Don't settle for less.

And if you're wondering, yes, my marriage came out the other side of the dry spell. But not because I shamed my partner, or myself. It happened because we both did the work— individually and together. And that, my dear, is how you ~~survive~~ thrive in a sexless relationship with your dignity and your sexy intact.

LESSON EIGHT

WHAT THE HELL IS A NARCISSIST, ANYWAY?

NARCISSISM. It's the turmeric of the psychological world these days. The word has become so ubiquitous it's practically a guest star in dinner conversations:

"My ex is a narcissist!"

"My boss? Total narcissist!"

But has narcissism really proliferated like avocado toast, or are we just overusing the term?

Before we diagnose literally half the population, let's take a moment to understand what narcissism truly is—and what it isn't. Because while narcissistic traits can charm us, frustrate us, or leave us reeling, only a small fraction of the population actually meets the criteria for Narcissistic Personality Disorder (NPD). Not to say your boss isn't one. Let's dive in.

NARCISSISM: THE SPECTRUM

Leave it to the romantic Greeks to create a myth about a beautiful hunter who was so entranced with his own image in a pool that he shunned all else—love, food, and drink. Which seems short-sighted to me, but whatever. Then he died, because . . . obviously.

Thus was born . . . narcissism. Coined by an English sexologist at the turn of the twentieth century, then Freud got a hold of it and BOOM. (Oh and back then? They declared it a sexual perversion. History lesson for the day!)

Soo . . . back from commercial break. Narcissism exists on a spectrum. At one end, we have *healthy narcissism*: a sprinkle of self-love that empowers us to chase dreams, ask for that promotion, or flirt with the hottie at the bar. It's adaptive and fuels ambition, confidence, and joy.

But at the extreme OTHER end lies Narcissistic Personality Disorder (NPD). This isn't just 'being full of yourself;' it's a diagnosable mental health condition that only trained professionals can identify, because it's tricky. Only about 1-2 percent of the world's population has true NPD.

Narcissism involves pervasive issues with empathy, intimacy, and self-regulation—traits that make relationships (and life) a battlefield. Think grandiosity, entitlement, and a lack of accountability—but with a secret ingredient: a hidden, fragile sense of self.

Here's the rub: most people we call narcissists don't meet the clinical definition. They're likely a-holes with emotional immaturity, not pathological narcissists. But the culture can amplify these traits and even encourage it! And for the record: malignant narcissism—the new coined phrase—is a syndrome comprising a mix of narcissism, antisocial behavior, sadism, and a paranoid outlook on life. I'll just leave that little morsel right there.

OKAY, WAIT . . . BUT WHY ARE NARCISSISTS SO MAGNETIC?

Narcissists are serious freakin' charmers. They're the life of the party, the ones who sweep you off your feet with grand gestures and audacious confidence. Their allure? An intoxicating mix of magnetism, ambition, and self-assuredness. But as the relationship deepens, their self-focus often takes center stage, leaving you feeling sidelined.

Sound familiar? That's because narcissists often attract their opposite: echoists. Echoists fear being a burden, over-accommodate, and shrink in the presence of a larger-than-life partner. It's a dynamic that can feel like a magnetic pull—and a trap.

Cinematic examples of narcissists—because it ain't always easy to spot one—include Cersei Lannister from *Game of Thrones*, the Evil Queen from *Snow White*, Don Draper from *Mad Men*, Walter White from *Breaking Bad*, and some celebrities who I can't name because they have more expensive lawyers than I do.

THREE RED FLAGS TO INDICATE THAT YOU MIGHT BE DATING A NARCISSIST

1. **The Self-Centered Superstar**: They boast about their greatness in everything *except* relationships. "I'm amazing at work, with friends, in life . . . but love? It's complicated." Translation: *I'm unwilling to do the emotional labor real relationships require.*
2. **The Trophy Spouse Seeker**: They're more interested in how you make them look than how you make them feel. Authentic love takes a backseat to appearances.
3. **The Fix-It Fantasy**: They hint that you're the one who needs to change. And if you dare suggest otherwise? *Gaslighting alert!* They deflect and deny.

THREE TIPS FOR COPING WITH A NARCISSISTIC PARTNER

1. **Hold the Line and Drop the Mic:** Narcissists will push, prod, and test, but your limits aren't a negotiation. Lay down the law on what's a *hard no*. They'll fight back, probably with the grace of a toddler denied Skittles, but stand firm. "No" isn't up for debate; it's a full sentence. Use it.
2. **Dodge the Blame Grenade:** Narcissists are pros at flipping the script. Don't let their gaslighting turn you into the villain of their soap opera. Their lack of empathy? That's *their* baggage, not yours. Return to sender, no forwarding address.
3. **Call in Your Backup Band:** You don't have to solo this gig. Find your crew—whether it's therapy, trusted friends, or a support squad—who can remind you that you're not crazy, you're just dealing with someone who is.

A FINAL THOUGHT

Narcissists are often driven by deep insecurity. Beneath their bravado lies a fragile self-image, constantly seeking validation. While this understanding can evoke empathy, it doesn't mean you have to endure the fallout of their behavior. It's not your responsibility to 'fix them.' Protect your peace, cherish your own self-worth, and remember: you deserve a partner who sees *you*, not just their reflection in your adoration.

Trying to come back from *oooh, I already dipped in that nasty pool?* Don't worry, love: we got you in Lesson 18.

LESSON NINE

LIBIDO LIMBO: WHEN DESIRE DOESN'T MATCH

THE DREADED MISMATCH. One of you wants it. The other doesn't. Or vice versa. And suddenly, what used to be easy feels like a tug-of-war where nobody wins.

Here's the deal: sexual desire ebbs and flows—it's normal. But when you're consistently out of sync, frustration brews. The good news? It's not a death sentence for your sex life. It's just a challenge that needs a little finesse, empathy, and strategy.

STEP 1: DROP THE BLAME, PICK UP THE MIRROR

Think of your relationship like two fish swimming in the same bowl—how do you move together instead of against each other?

Wanters: Their "no" isn't about you. Stress, exhaustion, hormones—desire is complex. Show appreciation beyond the bedroom.

Wanteds: Be honest about why you're not in the mood. Stress? Hormones? Feeling disconnected? A simple, "It's not no forever, just not now," can go a long way.

Empathy doesn't mean agreeing. It means seeing each other's perspective—and actually giving a damn.

STEP 2: BRING BACK THE SPARK (WITHOUT THE PRESSURE)

Desire doesn't just disappear—it gets buried under routine, stress, and responsibility. Time to dig it back up.

Recreate vacation mode. Late-night take-out dinners, a weekend just getting away, or even swapping childcare for uninterrupted time. Ditch the daily grind and make space for intimacy, even if for a few hours.

Focus on presence, not performance. Strip away the pressure for a specific outcome and just enjoy each other. Deep kisses, slow touches, hands intertwined—start there.

Inject novelty. Try something neither of you has done before. A sushi cooking class, an escape room, a horror movie —dopamine thrives on excitement, and so does attraction.

STEP 3: NEGOTIATE, DON'T CAPITULATE

Sexual harmony isn't about one person giving in—it's about meeting in the middle.

Define your 'yes,' 'no,' and 'maybe' zones. If one of you isn't up for full-on sex, what about a sensual massage? A slow makeout session? Listening to some hot jazz in the bath? Intimacy has layers.

Schedule sex. Unsexy? Maybe. Effective? Absolutely. It reassures the wanter and gives the wanted time to get in the right headspace.

Proactive "no's" with follow-ups. If it's not happening tonight, suggest a time when it will. "Not now, but let's plan something special this weekend." Simple. Considerate. Game-changer.

THREE KEYS TO LIBIDO HARMONY

Ask, don't assume. Instead of jumping to blame, ask, "What's going on for you?"

Prioritize quality over quantity. Maybe it's less frequent but better, more connected intimacy.

Keep talking. Silence breeds resentment. Keep the conversation open, honest, and shame-free.

The truth? The 'wanted' sets the tempo of intimacy. If that's you, own your power wisely. If you're the 'wanter' (as I once was), protect your self-esteem—find pleasure in your own body, too.

Mismatched libido isn't a crisis—it's an opportunity. When you navigate it with care, it deepens connection, strengthens partnership, and makes your sex life richer than ever. And isn't that the goal? To live sexily ever after—together.

LESSON TEN

IS LINGERIE A GIMMICK? WHY YOU DON'T NEED ITTY-BITTY LACY THINGS TO FEEL SEXY

Lingerie—the lacy little nothings sold as the ultimate shortcut to sex appeal. But is it a gimmick or a gateway to something deeper? Strip away the marketing, and what's left? Confidence? Power? Play? Let's untangle the silky straps of this one.

A BRIEF HISTORY: LINGERIE THROUGH THE AGES

The French gave us the word "lingerie," which evolved from *linge*, meaning linen. Originally, lingerie wasn't about seduction—it was about practicality. Picture women of centuries past, slipping out of heavy gowns into lighter undergarments to stay modest and hygienic. Fast forward to the twentieth century, and corsets gave way to more comfortable (and less injurious) alternatives thanks to pioneers like Lady Duff Gordon. Eventually, lingerie transformed into something we associate with allure, seduction, and, for some, playfulness.

Today, the sheer variety of lingerie can be overwhelming: baby dolls, bustiers, body stockings, tangas, garters—the list goes on and on. But the real question isn't what to wear; it's why we wear it.

LINGERIE AND THE SEXY FEEDBACK LOOP

The purpose of lingerie is deceptively simple: it's meant to make the wearer feel sexy. It's an external cue; a costume that lets us step into an erotic role. Put on red lace, and you become the temptress; slip into a black satin teddy, and you're a feline femme fatale. It's fun, yes, but here's the truth: you don't need lingerie to feel or be sexy.

Sexy isn't in the fabric—it's in you. The feedback loop starts within. When you feel sexy, you radiate it outward, and that confidence makes you even more attractive. If lingerie serves as a spark, by all means, embrace it. But the fire? That's your own.

THREE LESSONS FROM MIDLIFE LINGERIE WISDOM

In midlife, our relationship with lingerie—and ourselves—changes. What worked in our twenties might feel constraining or irrelevant now. I mean, I will never slip into some sexy butt floss again. So how do we strike the balance between comfort and allure? Here are three lessons to consider:

1. **Redefine What Sexy Looks Like for You**.
   Sexy doesn't mean 'the sex goddess in scarlet velvet' (unless you want it to). Maybe it's high-waisted boy-short panties that hug your curves just right. Maybe it's your partner's oversized button-down shirt, sleeves casually rolled up. Or maybe it's nothing but your favorite body lotion and a confident smile. Whatever makes you feel powerful and desirable—wear that. Ooo, yes. Wear that.
2. **Use Lingerie as a Tool, Not a Crutch**. Think of lingerie like dessert: tiramisu is delightful, but you wouldn't eat it every night. Use lingerie to spice things up when it feels exciting, not because you think

it's required. And remember: the best accessory isn't lace or silk, because that's just something you have to wash on delicate—it's your own authenticity.

3. **Dress for Yourself First**. Whether you're lighting candles for a solo bubble bath or planning a rendezvous with your partner, choose pieces that make you feel good. Feeling beautiful for yourself is just as important as dressing up for someone else. When you honor your own desires, you embody confidence—and that's irresistible.

THE PANDEMIC PAUSE AND POST-LINGERIE FREEDOM

Let's talk about the pandemic effect. Many of us ditched bras (and sometimes underwear) in favor of sweatpants. The result? We discovered a new kind of sexy—one that wasn't tied to satin or garters. This wasn't about rejecting lingerie but reclaiming comfort and authenticity.

I have a patient who did an experiment; a midlife woman who wore lingerie for seven consecutive nights. Her partner loved it, sure, but they also confessed she looked just as sexy in her polka-dot boxers. The takeaway? Your partner thinks you're sexy because you ARE sexy!

Lingerie is a prop, not the star of the show. If you love it, wear it. If not, skip it. Either way, the essence of your allure comes from your inner glow, your confidence, and your ability to embrace your authentic self.

A FINAL THOUGHT: LINGERIE DOESN'T MAKE YOU SEXY—YOU MAKE IT SEXY

So, rummage through your drawers. If those garters haven't seen daylight since your honeymoon, it might be time to say goodbye. If the tanga makes your poontanga itchy, launch it. Donate them, repurpose them, or toss them—but don't let them weigh you down. In midlife, you've earned the right to define your own sexy, without the gimmicks.

YOUR PLEASURE PRACTICE

Tonight, slip into something that makes you feel amazing. Maybe it's lingerie, maybe it's your thigh high stockings or button-down shirt, or maybe it's nothing at all. Strike a pose in front of the mirror and admire yourself. Sexy starts here.

LESSON ELEVEN

DON'T KILL MY VIBE! LET'S TALK SEX TOYS

WE'RE DELVING into a topic that deserves a seat at the grown-up table: **sex toys.** Whether you're partnered up, exploring new dynamics, or flying blissfully solo, it's time to add a little buzz to your bedroom (or wherever the mood strikes). Sex toys can enhance your sexual pleasure, deepen intimacy, and keep things spicy. And we love spicy.

THE MODERN TOOLKIT OF DESIRE

Sex toys are exactly that—tools. Just as you'd choose the right spatula for flipping pancakes or the perfect wrench to fix a leaky sink, the right toy can do wonders for scratching that particular itch. The best part? They're fun, accessible, and scientifically proven to help you explore your desires safely.

Let's address the biggest misconception: toys don't replace people; they enhance experiences. Whether you're sharing them with a partner or using them solo, toys are about creating pleasure, not competition. I mean, really, who can one up a device that buzzes at 15,000 vibrations per minute?

THE LONG, WINDING HISTORY OF SEX TOYS

Humans have been getting creative with pleasure for millennia. The oldest known dildo is 28,000 years old and carved from stone—proof that humans have always had an appreciation for, shall we say, self-love.

Vibrators, on the other hand, were initially invented in the 1880s as medical devices for women's 'hysteria.' Yes, my dear, a vibrator was once a prescription item, probably not covered by insurance though. Fast-forward to today, and we've traded in the clunky gadgets for sleek, ergonomic designs that can pulsate, rotate, and do everything short of write you poetry, although I'm sure that's in production.

HOW TO CHOOSE THE RIGHT TOY

Feeling overwhelmed by options? Let me guide you:

1. **Start simple.** If you're new to toys, opt for a basic vibrator or bullet designed for external clitoral stimulation. These are discreet, effective, and beginner-friendly.

2. **Consider your preferences.** Do you prefer internal stimulation? Try a G-spot vibrator or a dual-action rabbit. Curious about hands-free play? Explore suction toys or wearable vibes that deliver a whole new world of pleasure.

3. **Check the material.** Look for toys made of medical-grade silicone—they're body-safe, non-porous, and easy to clean. Avoid anything that feels overly cheap or contains questionable materials. Please don't order one that's ridiculously inexpensive and probably unethically made by Malaysian schoolchildren. That's not good for anyone.

4. **Know your intention.** Go for what sparks your curiosity—and like the princess and the frog, you may have to try a few before you find 'the one.'

TIPS FOR EVERY TYPE

- **For Long-Term Partners**: Toys can reignite intimacy and make the bedroom feel like new territory. Start with a vibrator designed for couples, like one with a remote control. Pass the remote to your partner for a playful dynamic. Advanced tip: take it out in public.
- **For New Partners**: Introducing toys early in a relationship might feel bold, but it's a great way to set the tone for open communication. Suggest something neutral like a vibrating cock ring—a fun, non-intimidating entry point for both of you.
- **For Solo Flyers**: Treat yourself! Consider investing in a high-quality clitoral suction toy or internal massager. The sky is the limit. Get one of everything! I once had a seventy-eight-year-old patient who had a huge collection and each one had a different man's name (Phil, Fred, Bob). Her fifty-year-old daughter was mortified. I thought she was a goddess. This was twenty years ago, and I guarantee you she died with a smile on her face. Point is, you're in charge of your pleasure, so go for gold.

KEEPING IT CLEAN (LITERALLY)

Your sex toys should bring you joy—not an unplanned trip to the gynecologist. Cleaning your toys after each use is non-negotiable.

Here's how:

1. **Use a toy cleaner or mild soap.** Avoid harsh chemicals; a gentle, fragrance-free cleanser works wonders.
2. **Air dry completely.** Avoid trapping moisture, which can lead to bacteria or fungus buildup.
3. **Store properly.** Keep your toys in a clean, dry place, ideally in a storage bag to avoid dust or contamination. Always check your toy each time before use to ensure that there are no rough spots and cutting edges. I've seen what happens when women don't do this: it involves stitches, let me just say.

SEX TOYS: TREND OR TIMELESS TOOL?

Toys are not a gimmick—they're a gateway to deeper self-awareness and richer intimacy. Whether you're using a toy for solo exploration, experimenting with a partner, or just trying something new, remember this: you make the toy sexy, not the other way around.

Don't shy away from the treasure chest of tools available to you. And if one toy doesn't vibe with you, try another. Think of it as sampling dessert—every taste is part of the fun.

YOUR PLEASURE PRACTICE

Because life is short, and pleasure is your birthright, pick one toy you've been curious about but hesitant to try. Order it online (hello, privacy!) and make a date to explore. Then, clean it lovingly and thank it for its service.

LESSON TWELVE

THE BLOOM BELOW: EMBRACING YOUR LADY GARDEN'S NATURE

OKAY, ladies. Let's have an honest conversation about something that's been unnecessarily burdening us for far too long: the scent of our lady bits. Stay with me here. Yes, our natural, beautiful, self-cleaning powerhouse. Too many of us hesitate to embrace our sensuality because of fears rooted in societal shame and marketing gimmicks. No more! (For movie rights: picture me here holding a large sword up in the air. I want it to be a big Joan of Arc-style saber.)

THE MYTH OF "FRESHNESS"

It's fascinating—or infuriating—how the scent of a woman's junk has become a topic of scrutiny while 'ball smell' doesn't even enter the cultural dialogue. From tight yoga pants to newfangled pH-balanced washes, we are inundated with messages that our natural scent needs fixing. Whooo-hoooo, spoiler alert: it doesn't.

Your genitalia is an intricate ecosystem. The vagina is a self-cleaning oven—it's designed to regulate its own pH, maintaining balance and cleansing itself. The slight musk or natural aroma you might notice? That's part of your body's healthy functioning; it can vary due to hormonal changes and it's never something to be ashamed of. Ever.

UNDERSTANDING YOUR BODY'S SYMPHONY

We're biologically equipped to detect changes in our own scent long before anyone else could. It's an evolutionary advantage; a way for your body to communicate with you. During different phases of your cycle, postpartum, or menopause, your scent will shift. This is a normal reflection of your body's remarkable adaptability. It does not mean the entirety of the grocery store can also smell you walking down Aisle 11.

To put it plainly, the warm, moist environment of your honey pot—akin to the lush Amazon—can sometimes result in a musty or slightly sour aroma. It's not a flaw. It's nature. What isn't normal? Scents reminiscent of a fish market or bread factory, which may indicate the need for medical attention. Trust your instincts and, if in doubt, consult your doctor.

THE CULPRITS OF MISUNDERSTANDING

Modern lifestyle factors, like tight clothing and synthetic fabrics, exacerbate discomfort and odor. Combine that with marketing ploys preying on insecurity, and it's no wonder so many women feel compelled to scrub themselves raw, which I have seen and it ain't pretty. But this overzealousness can backfire, disrupting your natural balance and causing irritation.

Remember: less is more. Your privates don't need an arsenal of fragranced products. In fact, many of these—from glitter-laden lotions to essential oils to scented toilet paper—can harm your sensitive skin.

PRACTICAL SELF-CARE

1. **Gentle Cleansing:** Stick to warm water. If you must use soap, choose an unscented, gentle option and avoid scrubbing. Freshen the landscaping, don't go in the house (AKA, stay on the outside to avoid vaginal irritation).
2. **Epsom Salt Baths:** A warm bath with plain Epsom salt can soothe irritation without disrupting your natural balance. Refrain from adding "Sultry Suds: Midnight Mango Mirage" bubble bath to your routine.
3. **Breathable Fabrics:** Opt for cotton underwear and looser clothing when possible to reduce heat and moisture buildup. Remove those tight workout pants after you're done with your sets.
4. **Refresh Naturally:** If you need a midday pick-me-up, try an unscented saltwater wipe, such as Boogie Wipes, which were invented for kids' snotty noses. But if it's good enough for a two-year-old's delicate smeller, it'll work with your hoo-ha.
5. **Cornstarch Powder:** In hot weather, a light sprinkle of cornstarch in your underwear can help absorb excess moisture. Stay away from talc products, which have been associated with ovarian cancer.

EMBRACE YOUR INNER SEXY

Confidence is magnetic. Knowing and embracing your body —its rhythms, scents, and all—is incredibly sexy. When you accept your female love temple as the masterpiece it is, you radiate a self-assurance that's irresistible to your partner and empowering for you.

A FINAL NOTE

Your coochie is a genius shape-shifter, a trickster, a marvel. She evolves with you through every stage of life. Don't let anyone—least of all a patriarchal marketing campaign—convince you otherwise. Tend to her with love and understanding, and she will reward you with comfort, health, and the freedom to fully embrace your sensuality. And yes, we can use the correct anatomical words, but I once won a contest in medical school for coming up with fifty synonyms for vomit, so I try to keep it real.

Ladies, let's rewrite the narrative. Your lady garden doesn't need to smell like a meadow; she needs to smell like you. And that, my dear, is glorious.

LESSON THIRTEEN

THIS IS WHAT SEX LOOKS LIKE... AFTER KIDS

I MEAN, let's get real. Parenthood changes everything. The thrill, spontaneity, and passion that once defined your relationship might now feel buried under piles of laundry, those shitty science fair projects, and sleepless nights. You might have even found a pacifier in your bra. But here's the secret: life after kids doesn't have to mean a life without intimacy. Let's unpack this together like a playdate in the park. Let me introduce you to a patient of mine (names have been altered).

STELLA'S STORY

Meet Stella. She's the mother of five children, ranging from preschoolers to teenagers. Stella came into my office dressed to kill but confessed that her sex life was nonexistent. "It's just not happening," she admitted.

She thought it would get better after the diapers, tantrums, and endless to-do lists, but here she was, still waiting for her libido to return.

Her story isn't unique. Parenthood often comes with a cocktail of exhaustion, shifting priorities, and an identity crisis. But here's the kicker: the real killer of post-kid intimacy is the word "should."

Bull should! Ban it from your vocabulary. There is no 'should' in sex or relationships—only what feels right for you and your partner in that moment.

WHY SEX SLOWS DOWN

1. **The First Year Blues**: Sleep deprivation, spit-up-stained clothes, and the relentless needs of a newborn can extinguish even the hottest flames. Most new parents hit pause on intimacy, which is natural and, I argue, even expected (although I have caught couples engaging in some postpartum play IN the hospital while recovering from birth). But I digress . . .

2. **The 'Middle Years' Myth**: Once kids start school, many parents expect their sex lives to rebound. But studies show couples with kids aged five to twelve report even less intimacy than new parents. There's endless things to do: ballet class, football, music lessons, car lines, and growing miniature humans. It's exhausting me just writing it!

3. **The Teenage Void**: Parents of teenagers are the least sexually active of all. The emotional and mental exhaustion of raising young adults, combined with middle age fatigue, often takes a toll. Plus, many parents struggle with how to be a role model sexually for their teens, because if we're thinking about it? They're thinking about it.

DIAGNOSING THE PROBLEM

- **Priorities**: When was the last time you put yourself first? You can't pour from an empty cup, yet many moms try. Prioritizing your needs is not selfish; it's essential. You would tell this same thing to your adult children some day!

- **Time**: Finding time for intimacy doesn't mean booking elaborate date nights. It means carving out small, meaningful moments to reconnect. Even hand holding while going to sleep can be intimate. We humans crave touch.
- **Fatigue**: Are you sleepy or soul-drained? Physical exhaustion is one thing; emotional depletion is another. Addressing your kind of fornication fatigue is key to reigniting desire.
- **Identity Crisis**: Becoming a parent often overshadows other parts of your identity. Can you be a 'good' mom and also rock a riding crop? (Yes. Yes, you can.)Reclaiming the 'you' that existed before kids is a powerful way to reconnect with your sexuality.

THREE TIPS FOR SPICY SEX AFTER KIDS

1. **Sex-Proof Your Home**
   - Thin walls? Invest in a sound machine. Creepy kids sneaking into your room? Use a series of baby gates or set boundaries for sleepovers.
   - Create a sacred space for intimacy, free from interruptions. Paul Newman and Joanne Woodward turned a closet in their home into a "fuck hut" so it was private from the rest of the family (their name, not mine, although it is fantastic).
2. **Rediscover Desire**
   - Your body and mind have changed since becoming a parent. Explore new fantasies, listen to erotica while doing chores, or watch something that excites you besides *Peppa Pig*.

What turned you on at twenty-five may not work at forty—and that's okay.

3. **Steal Moments**
   - Forget grand gestures. Intimacy can be five minutes of undivided attention: "How was your day?" *with* eye contact. Send a flirty text or a heartfelt note. It's the small, consistent sparks that rekindle the fire.

THE TAKEAWAY

Sex after kids doesn't have to be a casualty of parenthood. Prioritize yourself for real, steal moments for intimacy, and remember: you're not *just* a parent/grandparent and you don't have to suffer your sexy time to be one. You're still a vibrant, sensual, pleasure-deserving human being. By rekindling your connection with yourself and your partner, you're not only improving your relationship—you're modeling healthy self-love for your kids. Just ask Newman and Woodward's kids what they thought when they discovered their parents' love shack.

Throw 'should' out with the bathwater! Take a deep breath of longing and let's get back to living sexily ever after.

LESSON FOURTEEN

THIS IS WHAT SEX LOOKS LIKE AFTER... DIVORCE

AH, DIVORCE. THE BIG 'D,' or any breakup, isn't just a split; it's an identity shift. It's the end of a version of you that revolved around 'us.' But here's the reframe: divorce isn't a dead end; it's a diversion—a chance to reroute and rediscover your inner sexy.

WHY DIVORCE DISRUPTS YOUR SEXY

1. **Emotional Erosion:** A toxic partner or loveless dynamic chips away at confidence, often long before the actual breakup.
2. **Identity Crisis:** The life you built together—the plans and the dreams—vanishes. What's left can feel unfamiliar and intimidating.
3. **Social Whiplash:** Splitting assets, seeing your ex's new fling on Instagram, and answering "Why did you break up?" can make you want to hide under the covers forever.

Yet within the rubble of the old lies the foundation for something new: a sexier, freer you.

FROM DIVORCE TO DIVERT: A MINDSHIFT

The word "divorce" shares roots with "divert," which means to change direction. While divorce feels heavy and final, diverting is dynamic and full of possibilities. Embrace this reroute with intention:

1. **Cocoon Before You Fly**: Oh, it's so dang tempting: Jet to Bali! Swipe right on everyone! Go blonde! But before you set course for sunshine and Piña Coladas, or go platinum blonde, sit with your feelings. It is true science that if you face those feelings head on, they'll vanish faster. Most emotions can pass in ninety seconds if you point that wand at Voldemort and aim true. Write your story where you want: on paper, in the air, in the sand—the good, the bad, and the totally cringe-worthy. Processing the past is the first step to healing.

2. **Honor Your Libido Without Escapism:** Your libido is alive and well, but rushing into rebound flings or vodka-fueled nights won't heal you. You didn't intend to swipe right on a new case of ragin' gonorrhea. Instead, turn inward. Experiment with self-pleasure, sensual rituals, or new fantasies. Watch classic movies as a student of sensuality and reclaim your body as a source of joy—on your own terms. And, honey . . . PLEASE get a sexually transmitted infection screening at your nearby clinic.

3. **Redefine Sexy on Your Terms:** This is your blank slate. Want to explore tantra? Set firmer boundaries? Get new sex toys? Rediscover your turn-ons? Now's the time to rewrite your story (after Step 1) without anyone else's expectations

dictating the plot. It's a control-alt-delete on your whole sex life, so clear the cache and start fresh.

THREE PRESCRIPTIONS FOR POST-BREAKUP SEXY

1. **Date Yourself:** Who loves you most? You do! Take yourself out, dance like EVERYone's watching and you don't give a shit, and rekindle that spark with *you*. Fall in love with who you are today.
2. **Embrace Bold Confidence:** While I do love a makeover, skip anything dramatic looks-wise and instead get a dopamine hit by trying something new—killer shoes, a boudoir photo shoot, or a Bollywood class. Learn a new language or musical instrument. Small builds incite big confidence.
3. **Explore with Curiosity:** Your sexy is ageless. Dive into new fantasies, read or listen to loads of erotica (even old classics, such as Anaïs Nin), and see what ignites your curiosity and pleasure. Liberation starts with inquisition.

CLOSING THOUGHTS

Inner sexy isn't a mindset; it's a mind*shift*. A breakup isn't the end of your story; hell, no! It's a redirection. Think of it as a plot twist in your heroine's journey. And the best part? You're writing the next chapter, and it's going to be breathtaking.

LESSON FIFTEEN

THIS IS WHAT SEX LOOKS LIKE AFTER . . . A HYSTERECTOMY

You've decided to cast out your bitchy uterus—I'll call her Regina George for now—and NO one is talking about your sex life post-hysterectomy.

WHAT IS A HYSTERECTOMY, REALLY?

First, let's make sure we're speaking the same language for your next gyno visit:

- **Total Hysterectomy**: Removal of the uterus and cervix.
- **Total Hysterectomy with Bilateral Salpingo-Oophorectomy (BSO)**: Taking out the uterus, cervix, ovaries, and fallopian tubes—the whole shebang.
- **Partial (or Supracervical) Hysterectomy**: The uterus is removed, but the cervix stays.
- **Radical Hysterectomy**: This is the deep clean reserved for cancer treatment, removing tissue beyond just the uterus.

Why does this matter? Because understanding the specifics

of your surgery helps you navigate its physical and emotional aftermath—and why not sound like a total badass at your next appointment?

WHAT HAPPENS TO YOUR BODY (AND SEX LIFE) POST-HYSTERECTOMY?

Let's get real. A hysterectomy can be liberating for those plagued by heavy bleeding, pain, or fibroids. Imagine being free from the nightmare of Carrie-at-the-prom periods, or chronic discomfort during intimacy, or doubling over from stabbing cramps. For many women, the procedure is life-changing—and often, sex is better than ever.

But here's the flip side:

1. **Sensation Shifts**: If the cervix is removed, say goodbye to cervical orgasms. But no worries. You're not broken—you're just working with new equipment.
2. **Shortened Vagina**: In the case of a total hysterectomy, the vagina becomes a 'blind pouch,' potentially altering penetration depth. Most surgeons really work to avoid this being an issue.
3. **Hormonal Changes**: Removing the ovaries induces instant surgical menopause (it is, in essence, castration). This can lead to vaginal dryness, decreased libido, and a shift in how your body responds to stimulation. Also fixable!

YOUR INNER SEXY: POST-HYSTERECTOMY EDITION

So, what's next? How do you reclaim and reinvent your sexual self? Here are three tips to channel your inner sexy:

TAKE YOUR TIME

Despite the fact that you often go home the same or next day, healing after a hysterectomy is major. Nothing–NADA–in your vagina for at least six weeks. This prescription isn't just about following doctor's orders; it's about honoring your body's need to heal. 'Down there' is just so happy Regina is gone, but they need time to find their new normal.

- **Pro Tip**: If you have a partner, communicate with them. Let them know when you're ready (hint: not on their timeline). In the meantime, they can direct their energy toward housework—and maybe even surprise you with a clean house and a bangin' crock pot recipe.

EXPLORE NEW PLEASURES

Sex may not feel the same, but different doesn't mean worse. Reimagine intimacy:

- Focus on external stimulation (hello, dear clitoris!).
- Experiment with different positions to minimize discomfort.
- Try manual or oral techniques if penetration feels daunting at first.

Your body is a resilient powerhouse—treat it as a treasure map, not a loss.

EMBRACE LUBRICATION AND HORMONAL HELP

Dryness is common after ovary removal, but it's not insurmountable.

- Use high-quality lubricants and moisturizers designed for vaginal health. Beware of the pink tax! One of my favorite cheap tricks? A popped vitamin E capsule in the vagina.
- Discuss hormone replacement therapy (HRT) or non-hormonal options with your doctor to support both your libido and comfort.

RECLAIMING YOUR CONFIDENCE

A hysterectomy doesn't define your sexual vitality; it just asks you to rewrite the script. If your sexual pleasure feels diminished, seek new ways to connect—both with yourself and your partner. So many women tell me their sex life transcends because the bleeding/pain/cramping is a thing of the past! You're not the same woman you were pre-surgery, and that's okay. You're evolving, and so can your sex life. It's also okay to grieve a little bit for the removal of your uterus, because while Regina George can be a real bitch, she was a friend.

BOTTOM LINE

Adjusting to life after a hysterectomy is a process. Give yourself grace, advocate for your pleasure, and remember—your sexy isn't gone; it's just waiting for you to rediscover it. The mean girl is gone!

LESSON SIXTEEN

THIS IS WHAT SEX LOOKS LIKE AFTER...
CANCER

THE WORD alone can drain the room of its warmth. Cancer is not just unsexy—it's freakin' terrifying. And yet, for nearly 40 percent of all women, cancer will become a reality at some point in our lives. It's not just a number on a chart; it's a tidal wave that reshapes everything: our health, our emotions, our relationships, and, naturally . . . our inner sexy.

In the chaos of a diagnosis, treatment plans, telling friends and family, revised treatment plans, and survival, sex often falls to the bottom of the priority list. And who can blame us? Hair loss, surgical scars, nausea, pain, and fear of our mortality—none of these things scream "Oooh, I'm feeling so amazingly sensual."

But here's the truth no one talks about: reconnecting with your inner sexy after cancer isn't just about intimacy with others—it's about intimacy with yourself.

If treating hundreds of women with cancer has taught me one thing, it's that you can't skip the hard stuff. Although, damn, I wish we could, sister. I really wish we could. Grief, fear, anger—these emotions demand to be felt before we can reclaim our sense of self. And when we do, we'll discover a version of ourselves that is braver, deeper, and yes, SEXIER than ever before. Will it happen tomorrow? No, my angel. But it will happen if we hang in there. And if you're reading this and going through it . . . I already know you've got the stuff to *thrive* past cancer.

Here are three lessons to guide you on your journey:

LESSON ONE: REDEFINE SEXY ON YOUR TERMS

I once thought that sexy was sky-high bangs and ice-blue eyeshadow. And then it was ultra low-rise jeans and a crop tank top. The point is… sexy is not a one-size-fits-all descriptor. Maybe it used to mean silk lingerie and high heels. Maybe it still does! But post-cancer sexy could also look like a bold, bald head like one of the warrior Wakandan women from *Black Panther* (they are super sexy!), or a body softened by scars but fortified by survival. Sexy really just needs to be as simple as feeling at home in your own skin again.

Try this: Write a love letter to your body. Thank it for the battles it has fought and is still fighting. As women, we fight. We honor our resilience and rediscover the beauty in our imperfections. This act of self-compassion is the first step in seeing yourself—and showing yourself—as desirable.

LESSON TWO: PLEASURE IS MEDICINE

It's no secret that cancer wreaks havoc on the mind and body: fatigue, dryness, scarring, and hormonal changes can make sex feel daunting, even impossible. But pleasure—in all its forms—is healing. Orgasm floods the body with dopamine, oxytocin, and serotonin, the same feel-good chemicals that combat stress and pain.

Try this: Explore gentle, non-penetrative forms of intimacy. Massage, cuddling, or simply holding hands can reignite the connection with your partner. For solo exploration, invest in a quality vibrator or lubricant designed for sensitive skin.

Reclaim your pleasure, step by step. Don't let pressure from your partner expedite YOUR own healing sexual journey. A lot of women tell me that they engage past what they would like, "because he's a great guy, he's been so patient, blah, blah, blah."

He'll be okay, I promise you that! (Hand him a bottle of conditioner and tell him to hit the shower by himself, wink wink!) And if the shoe was on the other foot? You'd be compassionate and patient. Why do we expect less for ourselves?

LESSON THREE: BUILD AN INTIMACY TOOLBOX

Cancer can leave emotional scars that are deeper than the physical ones. Guilt, shame, or fear might make it hard to open up to a partner. Sometimes, partners themselves struggle to navigate the changes—they are just as scared as you are! I've even had women tell me that their *partners* shut off intimacy because they're terrified of hurting them, or that you will leave them. Building an intimacy toolbox can help you bridge that gap.

Try this: Your oncologist or cancer doctors are worried about your survival; they are piloting the rocket. They don't have the capacity to work through the environment around cancer, such as feeling sexy. And while many cancer centers offer wonderful adjuvants to therapy, such as talk therapy and even reiki, no one is quite on the forefront of sexual healing after cancer. Seek out a support group that specializes in cancer recovery *and* intimacy. These spaces can help you (and your partner) unpack the emotional weight of your experience. If therapy feels out of reach, start small. Find something that brings you pleasure, whether it's the perfect latte or the best soil for your garden (that wasn't intended to be a euphemism but let's go with it, shall we?). What is pleasurable about it? The smell? The taste? The touch? Senses = sensuality.

FINAL THOUGHTS: YOUR NEW YOU IS BEAUTIFUL

Cancer doesn't have to steal your inner sexy. Embracing this new chapter is an act of courage—one that makes you undeniably, powerfully desirable. *Sex and the City* addressed female sexuality with cancer nearly thirty years ago, but I want more! I want more movies and television shows delving into this issue, because with nine million new cancer cases in women each year, we could all use some relatable characters going through something similar and finding their sexy again. Remember: intimacy isn't just about hot orgasms (though we love that, too). It's about vulnerability, laughter, feeling, and joy. It's about finding new ways to say, "I'm still here. I'm still me. And I'm hella sexy in my own way."

LESSON SEVENTEEN

FANTASY OR FAIRYTALE? GREAT (S)EXPECTATIONS AND DISAPPOINTMENT

ONCE UPON A TIME, someone sold us a lie.

They told us that love should be effortless, passion should be endless, and sex should always be mind-blowing. They wrapped it in fairy tales, rom-coms, and glossy magazine headlines—until one day, we woke up and realized that real relationships don't come with background music or perfectly timed lighting.

THE FANTASY TRAP

Reality check: even the best love stories have plot holes.

From the moment we first heard bedtime stories about glass slippers and dashing princes, the seeds of fantasy were planted. Society whispered (and sometimes shouted) that our relationships should sparkle like a Disney movie glass slipper, that every kiss should curl toes, and that passion should burn hotter than a wood-fired pizza.

But here's the catch: fantasies, while delicious, can derail us. When we expect our partners (or ourselves) to deliver five-star, Michelin-level magic every day, we're setting up for disappointment. Worse, we lose sight of the real treasures: connection, resilience, and yes, even messy, leftover-hot-dog love.

STANDARDS VS. EXPECTATIONS

This isn't about settling. It's about shifting our lens. It's about recognizing the difference between **standards** (which keep us grounded) and **expectations** (which, when unchecked, can send us spiraling). It's about embracing the truth that some nights are champagne and fireworks, and others are takeout and sweatpants—and that both can be deeply satisfying.

Let's clarify two key terms that get tangled up in our hearts:

- **Standards** are the bedrock—non-negotiable deal breakers. These protect your dignity and keep you grounded. Think: mutual respect, physical safety, and kindness.
- **Expectations** are the clouds—stories we tell ourselves about how things *should* be. They're shaped by culture, media, and yes, that rom-com you watched last week. They can be exhilarating, but also treacherous.

Here's the golden rule: **Never lower your standards, but always check your expectations.**

THE FOOD ANALOGY

Not every meal is a five-star feast, and not every sexual encounter will be a symphony. Some nights, it's Michelin-starred magic; others, it's lukewarm mac and cheese. The same goes for relationships. Unrealistic expectations rob us of the joy of good-enough moments—moments that nourish us in ways we often overlook.

TIPS TO MANAGE EXPECTATIONS

Managing Sexual Expectations: Fantasy vs. Reality

1. **Let Go of the "Highlight Reel" Sex:** Sex isn't a perfectly lit, slow-motion, sweat-free montage. It's real, raw, sometimes awkward, sometimes mind-blowing. Let go of the idea that every encounter has to be peak-level passion. Some nights are all fireworks, others are just a warm glow—and both are valuable.

2. **Stop Measuring Sex by Frequency:** More sex doesn't automatically mean better sex. Instead of focusing on how *often* it happens, shift your mindset to *how connected* you feel—before, during, and after. A few deeply intimate moments are worth more than a dozen disconnected ones.

3. **Pleasure Isn't Just About the Finish Line:** If the goal is always orgasm, you're missing half the fun. Enjoy the slow build, the teasing, the sensation of touch without racing to the end. When you stop treating sex like a task to complete, it becomes an experience to savor.

4. **Your Libido Is Not Broken—It's Evolving**: Desire shifts throughout life. Stress, hormones, routine, and emotional connection all play a role. Instead of panicking when your libido changes, get curious. What excites you *now*? What turns you *off*? Treat your sexuality as something fluid, not fixed.

5. **Passion Needs Space to Breathe:** Whether you're single or partnered, routine is the enemy of desire. Change up where and how you experience pleasure—try a different setting, a new way of touching, or simply take a break from autopilot sex. Passion isn't lost; it's just buried under predictability. Dig it out.

THE PLEASURE PRACTICE

Write down one expectation you're ready to let go of and one standard you'll fiercely protect. Remember, perfection is truly the enemy of pleasure, and reality—when embraced—can be even sexier than fantasy.

Until next time, stay grounded, stay sexy, and for goodness' sake, let yourself enjoy the macaroni and cheese. And she lived sexily ever after. . . the end.

LESSON EIGHTEEN

FROM NARCISSIST NIGHTMARE TO SENSUAL SUPERHERO

Narcissists don't just drain your energy—they hijack your sensuality, rewriting the script of what you deserve, what you should tolerate, and how much of yourself you should give away. If you've survived a narcissistic relationship, whether in or out of the bedroom, it's time to reclaim what's yours: your power, your pleasure, and your unapologetic self-worth.

This is your guide to getting past them—not just leaving, but healing so deeply that they could never touch you again.

STEP ONE: CUT THE CORD—FOR REAL THIS TIME

Leaving a narcissist isn't just physical—it's mental, emotional, and chemical. Trauma bonds are real. The pull to seek validation from them? Also real. But that chapter is over. Here's how to make sure you actually close the book:

- **Go full "No Contact" (or as close as possible).** Block them. No social media stalking. No checking to see if they miss you. They don't. And even if they did, it wouldn't change anything. No contact. Period.

- **Scrub their presence from your life.** Delete texts, unfollow their friends, get rid of the playlist you made together. Narcissists live in the emotional residue they leave behind—wipe them out.

- **Expect the hoover.** They will try to pull you back in. Maybe with guilt, maybe with a love bomb, maybe with a crisis they suddenly need you for. Do not fall for it. Their "change" is as real as a reality show romance.

STEP TWO: DETOX THEIR VOICE FROM YOUR HEAD

The narcissist's greatest trick? Making you doubt yourself. Maybe they called you "too sensitive," made you feel undesirable, or had you walking on eggshells. Time to burn those old scripts.

- **Rewrite the narrative.** List three things they made you believe about yourself that were absolute lies—then rewrite the truth. Example:
- "I was too much" → "I am powerful and intense in the best way."
- **Purge their approval-seeking patterns.** Did they train you to over-explain, apologize for existing, or crave validation? Notice those habits and break them. Practice saying "No." Walk away without explaining yourself. Exist without permission.
- **Turn their insults into your superpower.** If they mocked your emotions, celebrate your deep-feeling self. If they belittled your independence, lean hard into your solo strength. Whatever they tried to diminish? Double down on it.

STEP THREE: REBUILD YOUR SENSUALITY FROM THE INSIDE OUT

Narcissists distort intimacy, making it transactional, performative, or just another power game. Now, it's time to take back your pleasure—without anyone else's approval.

- **Reconnect with your body.** Dance naked in your room. Sleep sprawled across the bed. Take long showers just to feel yourself. Remind your body that it is yours, and only yours.

- **Reclaim touch as pleasure, not obligation.** Whether it's self-massage, trying new fabrics against your skin, or taking up a movement practice like yoga or pole dancing—touch should feel good again. No pressure, no performance. Just sensation.

- **Explore your desires—on your terms.** Not what they wanted. Not what you thought would make them stay. What do you crave? Read erotic literature. Watch something sensual. Fantasize freely. Your pleasure, your rules.

STEP FOUR: RELEASE WITHOUT FORGIVENESS (IF THAT'S WHAT YOU NEED)

Forget the Hallmark version of healing—closure isn't always about forgiveness. You don't have to "understand" them, you don't have to "let it go," and you sure as hell don't have to excuse the damage they did.

- **Release the idea that you needed their love.** You needed love, yes—but not theirs. Their "love" was a weapon, not a gift. You were not wrong for wanting love. But now, you get to seek it elsewhere —starting with yourself.

- **Stop replaying the "What If" fantasy.** There is no version of this story where they finally see your worth. No alternate ending where they change. The only ending that matters is you walking away and never looking back.

- **Let the anger fuel you—then let it burn out.** Rage is useful. It's a catalyst. Let it remind you why you left. But don't let it be your forever state. Move from anger into power. Power into peace. Peace into pleasure.

PLEASURE PRACTICE: WRITE A SENSUAL PERMISSION SLIP

Narcissists make you doubt what you deserve. So tonight, write yourself a sensual permission slip.

Start with: "I give myself permission to..."

Examples:

"I give myself permission to take up space, to be loud, to be soft, to experience deep pleasure without shame, to be loved fully and freely."

Write it. Say it out loud. Feel it sink in. Because this—this return to your power—is what makes you a Sensual Superhero.

THE LAST WORD (AND IT'S YOURS)

Escaping a narcissist isn't just about leaving a toxic relationship—it's about rediscovering the parts of you they tried to erase. It's about knowing you are desirable, magnetic, untouchable in your own energy.

You don't need their validation. You never did.

Your next chapter? It's going to be electric. Sensual. Unapologetic. And sexy as hell.

LESSON NINETEEN

STOP LETTING THOSE HANDCUFFS GO TO WASTE—LET'S GET KINKY!

You watched *Fifty Shades* and chortled (love that word). Maybe you got a set of handcuffs for a Halloween sexy cop kind of costume or as a gag gift from your bestie at the office. Sometimes, you find them in your bedroom nightstand shoved behind old magazines, chargers, and some lotion that you swore you would use nightly for your dry skin. But hey, you've kept them! You didn't donate them to . . . not sure where you could donate handcuffs to? Maybe the local theater for a re-staging of *Les Mis*? Somewhere deep down, didn't you always suspect they *might* come in handy?

Here's the thing: exploring kink, fetish, and fantasy doesn't mean signing up for an underground dungeon club (though, if you're curious, they're surprisingly well-organized). It's about curiosity and giving yourself permission to play. Let's break it down, laugh a little, and maybe—just maybe—turn those handcuffs into more than an inside joke.

KINK, FETISH, AND FANTASY: WHAT'S WHAT?

To navigate the terrain, we need a map. Here's your quick and dirty guide, no quizzes later, promise:

- **Kink:** Kink is the broadest category—think of it as the buffet of sexuality. It's everything outside the standard dinner-and-a-movie script. A kink could be light spanking, dirty talk, or pretending you're the last two humans on Earth trying to repopulate during a zombie apocalypse. Or . . . playing the actual zombies, if that's enticing to you.

The beauty of kink? It's deeply personal and gloriously weird. Your kink might be silk scarves and scented candles; someone else's might be watching Zillow listings while wearing four-inch heels. (Yes, house hunting can be kinky. Who knew escrow could be so erotic?)

- **Fetish:** Fetishes zero in on specific objects or actions that are essential for arousal. Shoes, latex, feet—fetishes transform the seemingly mundane into the utterly thrilling. If kink is the spice rack of sexuality, a fetish is your go-to bottle of hot sauce.

And yes, the *DSM-5* (the psychiatrist's encyclopedia) calls fetishes "paraphilias," which sounds suspiciously like a Harry Potter spell. But don't let the jargon scare you. Fetishes are just another way of saying, "This thing turns me on, and I'm not mad about it."

If you are wondering if it's a fetish, there's probably an Only Fans account dedicated to it.

- **Fantasy:** Ah, fantasies—the sexiest daydreams your brain can conjure. Want to star in your own steamy pirate adventure? Or reenact that sketch scene from *Titanic* (minus the iceberg)? Fantasies are your personal playground, where anything goes, and no one has to know.

Bonus: Fantasies don't have to involve props, costumes, or a Pinterest board. I mean, they can, and that can be super fun to plan out, because who doesn't love to plan a scene? And get creative, let those juices flow (all of them). Tired of the ol' boss/secretary? Do sexy judicial confirmation hearings that turn randy. Or maybe your partner pretends to be an artificial intelligence program and they're texting you back . . . but it turns sexy. But the old standards work great, also. Fantasies are great because they're portable, private, and endlessly customizable.

HOW TO DIVE IN WITHOUT LOSING YOUR COOL

START LIGHT: THE FOREPLAY OF KINK

Kink is like salsa—start mild before you go full ghost pepper. A silk blindfold or a feather tickler is a perfect way to test the waters. These are available online for a host of reasons (cat toys, for one, have feathers on them and Jeff Bezos will be none the wiser about your ulterior motives). Maybe a gentle spanking or playful restraint. Use what you already have— that's where it gets fun! Not ready for a ball gag? Try a satin scarf first. (Pro tip: scarves also double as chic accessories. No one will know your neckwear moonlights as bondage gear.)

And if you try something and hate it? Congratulations! As my mama always said to me at the dinner table, "You don't have to like it, but you do have to try it."

Now I'm wondering if she was really talking about that casserole or giving me future midlife advice? Note to self: ask Mom. Point is, not every experiment will light your fire, but the cat will *love* that feather toy. Trust me.

COMMUNICATE. (WITHOUT MAKING IT WEIRD.)

Sharing a kink or fantasy can feel like stepping into the spotlight wearing nothing but your birthday suit. Start small: "I saw this thing on TV, and it looked . . . interesting."

Or, "What do you think about trying something new?"

Gauge your partner's response. If they're intrigued, great! If they're horrified, remember: that's about them, not you. Some people need time to adjust, and others might never share your particular taste. Either way, you've opened a conversation, and that's sexy in itself. If you're solo, then all the better! The stage is all yours and you are the freakin' star!

FANTASIES: YOUR EROTIC CHOOSE-YOUR-OWN-ADVENTURE.

Man, I loved those books as a kid. Want to try something truly daring? Let your imagination run wild. Get a sexy nom de plume, write your fantasy down, share it with a partner, or just keep it for yourself. Sometimes when you have your own Sasha Fierce avatar name, you can break out of your old bounds. (Mine is Lila Lovewell.) Literally any AI program can help you do this as well, if you don't fancy yourself a Jude Devereux. Now I wonder if that's her real name. You can act it out, talk about it, or let it simmer in your mind like a sexy secret.

And remember: there's NEVER ANY judgment in fantasy land. Whether you're dreaming of being rescued by a fire-fighter or leading a Viking raid, it's all part of the fun.

THE FINE PRINT: SAFETY AND CONSENT

Before you dive into kinkier waters, keep a few ground rules in mind:

- **Consent is sexy:** Always make sure everyone's on board with the plan.
- **Safety first:** Some activities, like breath play or bondage, can be risky. Research, communicate,

and never go solo on anything that could be dangerous or you'll end up an urban legend.

- **Legality matters:** Believe it or not, necrophilia (yep, you read that right) is still legal in some US states (looking at you, Louisiana). But just because you *can* doesn't mean you *should*. Stay within the bounds of the law, and remember: no kink is worth jail time. Seriously, people. Mug shots are never flattering.

PERMISSION TO PLAY

You've waited long enough to start exploring. Whether it's breaking out the handcuffs, shopping for lingerie, or simply letting your imagination roam, give yourself permission to embrace the fun, the silly, and the downright sexy.

Midlife is the perfect time to rewrite the script and stop holding back. Those handcuffs? They're not just a metaphor. They're an invitation to get curious, get playful, and—yes— get a little kinky. Meeee-owww.

LESSON TWENTY

GRATITUDE SEX—WHY BEING THANKFUL IS THE NEW SEXY

The word "gratitude" might feel overused, like oat milk lattes or CBD gummies. But here's the kicker: just like those trends, gratitude actually works. (I mean, ask my digestive system!) And if your love life has been gathering dust—whether due to stress, work, partners, kids, or sheer social media exhaustion—practicing gratitude might just rekindle the spark.

You heard me right. Gratitude can make sex hotter. Science says so. It boosts mood, lowers stress, improves emotional connection, and—get this—can increase libido. So if you're feeling 'meh' in the bedroom, it's time to tap into the power of authentic appreciation. Let's break it down into three actionable paths for partners, new lovers, and solo adventurers.

THE SCIENCE OF GRATITUDE (AND WHY IT'S SO DAMN SEXY)

Gratitude isn't just a feel-good buzzword. Studies show it lowers blood pressure, decreases anxiety, and even fosters self-acceptance and personal growth. When applied to relationships, it builds what researchers call "sexual communal strength"—the willingness to meet your partner's sexual and emotional needs. In short, when you appreciate each other, you're more likely to light each other up.

And it's not about keeping score. "Thanks for unloading the dishwasher" doesn't need to be repaid tit-for-tat (pun intended). True gratitude—like true foreplay—comes from a place of sincerity, not obligation.

WHY GRATITUDE WORKS IN THE BEDROOM

Gratitude changes your brain. Literally. It increases dopamine —the same feel-good chemical behind infatuation and pleasure. By thanking what you love, you prime your brain for connection, warmth, and . . . fireworks. As humans, we long to feel appreciated.

A CASE STUDY: FROM BLAH TO BLUSH-WORTHY

One of my midlife patients, we'll call her Seraphina Lux, self-described her relationship as "blah." She was skeptical of gratitude. But she tried it, because our motto is "you don't have to like it, but you really should try it." She started small, texting her partner simple thank yous for teeny things they did, like closing the garage door. The response was instant, and their mutual appreciation snowballed. Within weeks, they weren't just grateful—they went from blah to beguiling.

Gratitude isn't magic, but it's damn close. And when practiced authentically, it's the gift that keeps on giving to ourselves and others—in and out of bed.

So, how do we weave this into our daily lives (and beds)? Here's your guide.

Make gratitude foreplay a ritual. Before jumping into bed, take a moment to share *one* thing you appreciate about your partner (or yourself, if flying solo). It can be as deep as "I love how safe I feel with you" or as simple as "Your laugh makes my day." Verbal appreciation creates emotional closeness—and emotional closeness turns up the heat.

Say thank you *after* sex. Post-sex gratitude is underrated. Instead of rolling over and grabbing your phone, acknowledge the moment. "That was incredible." "I love how you touched me." "Damn, I needed that." It reinforces connection and makes your partner (or yourself) feel valued in and out of the bedroom.

Turn daily gratitude into *desire*. Gratitude doesn't just belong in the bedroom—cultivate it all day long. Compliment your partner on something non-sexual, and watch how it spills over into intimacy. "I admire how patient you are with the kids" can translate to "I see you, I value you"—which is sexy as hell.

Rewire your brain with a "Sexy Gratitude List". Make a list of three things you love about your body. Keep it raw, real, and *not* perfection-focused. "I love the way my hips move when I walk" is just as valid as "I love how my body lets me experience pleasure."

Express gratitude physically. Instead of just *saying* thank you, show it. A lingering touch when they pass by, a squeeze of the hand, a slow kiss at the end of the day. Physical appreciation reinforces emotional gratitude and reminds you both that affection doesn't have to lead to sex—but it sure can.

Write a love letter to your sexuality. Take five minutes to write a letter to your sexual self. Thank her for evolving, for discovering new desires, for enduring the highs and lows of intimacy. Acknowledge her resilience and power. Re-reading this when you're feeling disconnected from yourself can be a game-changer.

PLEASURE PRACTICE: THE 30-SECOND GRATITUDE EXPERIMENT

Tonight, before bed, close your eyes and think of one thing—big or small—that you're grateful for about your body or your love life. Maybe it's your hands, the way they feel against your skin. Maybe it's a specific memory of pleasure. Maybe it's simply that you're here, open to experiencing more joy. Let that gratitude settle into your body, and notice what shifts.

Gratitude isn't about *settling* for what you have—it's about *savoring* it. And in sex, as in life, that makes all the difference.

FINAL TIP: GRATITUDE IS SEXY, BUT IT HAS TO BE REAL

If your gratitude feels forced or snarky ("Thanks for <u>finally</u> putting the toilet seat down"), it'll backfire. Authenticity is key. Start small. Be specific. Even with yourself. "Thanks, little finger, for always sticking up straight when I drink tea." And let it grow naturally. Before you know it, you'll be living—and loving—sexily ever after.

LESSON TWENTY-ONE

MISSIONARY... WHY YOU SHOULDN'T TAKE IT OFF THE TABLE (OR BED) JUST YET

Ah, missionary—the position that's been both unfairly maligned and quietly adored. It's often dismissed as vanilla, but much like a classic film or a perfectly tailored little black dress, missionary has *range*. It's intimate, versatile, and shockingly easy to upgrade.

At its core, missionary is about connection—skin to skin, face to face, breath against breath. It allows for deep intimacy, emotional engagement, and, with the right tweaks, some of the best pleasure potential out there. So before you file it under "basic," let's talk about why it deserves a spot in your rotation.

FUN FACT: WHY "MISSIONARY?"

Legend has it that the term "missionary position" originated from prudish Christian missionaries who deemed it more civilized than other animalistic options. In reality, the term only surfaced in the mid-twentieth century, likely the result of a mistranslation. Despite its dubious etymology, missionary has endured as a staple of human connection.

Some options for rebranding: lovers' lock, face-to-face fiesta, the vanilla thrilla'. Ok, we'll keep working on it.

WHY KEEP IT IN THE MIX?

Here's the kicker: missionary works. Studies show that women often achieve orgasm more frequently in this position due to its potential for direct clitoral stimulation and the emotional connectivity it fosters.

It's also incredibly versatile. Whether you're looking for deep intimacy, full-body closeness, or just a go-to that doesn't require the flexibility of a gymnast, missionary delivers. And let's not forget—it's great for same-sex couples too, proving that this classic position isn't just about tradition, but about maximizing pleasure in a simple, effective way.

But even the best classics need a remix. Here's how to make it work for you.

FIVE WAYS TO MAKE MISSIONARY WORK FOR YOU

1. ADJUST THE ANGLES FOR MAXIMUM PLEASURE

Not all missionary is created equal. Small adjustments can take it from *meh* to *mind-blowing*.

- **The Pillow Trick:** Placing a pillow under the hips changes the angle, making penetration feel deeper and more direct. This is especially helpful for increasing clitoral stimulation.
- **Leg Positioning:** Keep legs flat for a close, intimate fit. Bend the knees to open up access. Elevate the legs over shoulders for an even deeper stretch and intensity.
- **Side-Slip Variation:** Shift slightly so the top partner's torso is angled more to one side, changing friction points and creating new sensations.

2. ELEVATE THE SENSORY EXPERIENCE

Missionary is a perfect position for full-body connection—use it to heighten pleasure through the senses.

- **Eye Contact:** It's optional, but if you can hold a gaze without laughing or looking away, it can create an intense connection. A few seconds of deep eye contact before closing your eyes makes all the difference.
- **Breath Syncing:** Matching breathing rhythms naturally relaxes the body and can heighten arousal. Try inhaling and exhaling together—it sounds small, but it builds intimacy fast.
- **Slow It Down:** Instead of treating missionary as a means to an end, focus on slowing movements, exploring touch, and being fully present.

3. BRING IN TOYS FOR NEXT-LEVEL SENSATION

Missionary is the perfect position for integrating external stimulation without disrupting the moment.

- **Use a Small Vibrator:** A slim toy placed between bodies can enhance sensation for both partners.
- **Try a Vibrating Ring:** A cock ring with vibration can add a new layer of stimulation without any effort.
- **Experiment with Temperature:** Ice cubes on the skin, a warm massage candle, or a cooling gel can amplify sensation in subtle but exciting ways.

4. EXPLORE HANDS-ON PLEASURE

One of missionary's best features? Easy access for extra stimulation.

- **Hand Play:** Whether it's touching your own body, guiding a partner's hand, or incorporating gentle pressure on different areas, missionary allows for easy exploration.
- **Intracourse (Non-Penetrative Play):** This position is great for thigh grinding, outercourse, or slow teasing movements that don't rely solely on penetration.
- **Pressure Points:** Applying gentle or firm pressure on hips, thighs, or even gripping hands together can intensify arousal without changing the rhythm.

5. TIPS FOR THE SOLO GAL

Missionary isn't just for partnered play—it's also one of the best positions for self-pleasure.

- **Change Up Your Positioning:** Lying on your back with bent knees can enhance sensation and allow for easier access with your hands or toys. Try experimenting with different angles to find what works best for you.
- **Make It a Full-Body Experience:** Use this time to engage all your senses—soft blankets, a heated toy, a slow build-up. Instead of rushing, focus on the *feeling* of touch and connection with yourself.

VANILLA, WITH EXTRA TOPPINGS (VARIATIONS TO SPICE THINGS UP)

- **The Magic Bullet**: Legs straight up or over shoulders. A bit more demanding but worth the effort.
- **The Quesadilla**: Bodies pressed completely together. Maximum skin contact for those who crave closeness.
- **Thigh Play**: Intercourse isn't the only option—this position lends itself to creative exploration, like "'intracourse'" or using hands and toys.

THE BOTTOM LINE

Missionary isn't a relic of the past—it's a foundation to build on. By tweaking angles, incorporating sensation, and focusing on connection, this so-called "vanilla" position transforms into something rich, deep, and endlessly customizable.

Don't write it off. Remix it. Play with it. And remember, the classics never go out of style.

LESSON TWENTY-TWO

LUBE, GLORIOUS LUBE! YOUR GUIDE TO SLIDING INTO PLEASURE

Let's talk about one of life's greatest unsung heroes: lube. Yes, lube—the silky, slick sidekick that has been saving sex lives for eons yet is often overlooked or, worse, stigmatized. It's time to change that. Whether you're rediscovering long-term passion, embarking on a new romantic adventure, or indulging in solo pleasure, lube isn't just a backup plan—it's a game-changer.

THE SCIENCE OF WETNESS

A quick refresher on biology: the vagina doesn't have traditional lubrication glands like your eyes or mouth. Instead, moisture comes from blood flow. When aroused, nitric oxide dilates blood vessels, allowing fluids to pass through the vaginal walls and mix with water, proteins, and skin cells to create that glorious glide.

But here's the reality check: estrogen fuels this process, and as estrogen naturally declines (hello, perimenopause and beyond), so can natural lubrication. Add in certain medications—antihistamines, antidepressants, even birth control—and you might find dryness crashing the party uninvited. That's where lube comes in, ready to smooth things over and restore the pleasure you deserve.

WHY LUBE IS NON-NEGOTIABLE

Lube isn't just about reducing friction. It enhances sensation, eliminates discomfort, and, let's be honest, makes everything *better*. Yet so many of us hesitate to reach for it. Why? Outdated myths, shame, or the mistaken belief that using lube means your body is "failing" you.

Let's be clear: needing or wanting lube is perfectly normal and ridiculously smart. It's not a sign of aging, dysfunction, or a lack of attraction—it's a tool for maximizing pleasure. And who doesn't want that?

YOUR LUBE TOOLBOX: CHOOSING THE RIGHT ONE

Not all lubes are created equal, and picking the right one can make all the difference.

Water-Based Lubes

- **Pros:** Universal, safe with condoms and toys, easy to clean.
- **Cons:** Can dry out quickly, requiring reapplication.
- **Best for:** All-purpose use, spontaneous moments, and beginners.

Silicone-Based Lubes

- **Pros:** Long-lasting, silky texture, waterproof (yes, shower sex approved).
- **Cons:** Not compatible with silicone toys, can feel a bit slicker than some prefer.
- **Best for:** Post-menopausal dryness, marathon sessions, and water play.

Oil-Based Lubes

- **Pros:** Rich, creamy, and long-lasting.
- **Cons:** Not safe for condoms, may disrupt vaginal pH.
- **Best for:** Solo play, massages, and those in monogamous relationships where condoms aren't needed.

Specialty Lubes

- **Warming/Cooling:** Adds sensation but proceed with caution—what sounds fun can sometimes feel like a *chemical warfare* experiment.
- **Flavored:** Playful for oral, but watch for sugar content, which can disrupt vaginal health.
- **Moisturizing:** Hybrid lubes that work for both intimacy and daily hydration (great for vaginal dryness).

FIVE WAYS TO MAKE LUBE WORK FOR YOU

1. **Make Lube Part of Foreplay**. Lube isn't just for the main event. Treating application as a sensual ritual instead of a clinical necessity changes the game. Warm it between your fingers, apply it with intention, and make it part of the experience.
2. **Keep It Accessible. (Like, Right There.)** The last thing you want in the heat of the moment is to rummage through drawers or sprint to the bathroom. Keep a small, elegant bottle on the nightstand, in a bedside drawer, or tucked into your travel bag so it's always within reach.
3. **Upgrade Solo Sessions with the Right Lube.** For the solo adventurers, lube can make all the

difference. Try a thicker, moisturizing lube for extended play or a silicone-based lube if you don't want to reapply. Think of it as self-care—because it is.

4. **Experiment with Sensation (But Know Your Limits.)** Curious about warming lubes? Cooling sensations? Try a *tiny* amount first. What's labeled as "tingling" on the bottle might feel more like a five-alarm fire in practice. When in doubt, test before you dive in.

5. **Don't Just Use Lube—Hydrate Like a Pro.** For daily vaginal hydration, puncture a vitamin E capsule and apply it internally before bed. It's a simple, cost-effective way to keep things supple without the overpriced "feminine moisture" creams.

THE FINAL SLIDE: WHY LUBE IS A MUST-HAVE

Lube is not just a "fixer" for dryness—it's an enhancer of pleasure, intimacy, and self-love. Whether you're smoothing the way for a new adventure, rediscovering familiar territory, or flying solo, it belongs in your sensual toolkit.

No guilt, no stigma—just the ultimate invitation to more glide, more comfort, and more pleasure. Because you, my dear, deserve nothing less.

LESSON TWENTY-THREE

WHY INTIMACY COMES WITH IRRITANTS—CAUSES, CURES, AND QUICK RELIEF

Ah, intimacy. The warmth of connection, the fireworks of passion—and sometimes, the unwelcome encore of post-sex irritation. We're diving into the not-so-glamorous reality of the 'fire ant' sensation that can follow even the most satisfying romp. This isn't about emotional gripes; we're talking about literal physical discomfort. So let's unpack why it happens and how to banish it so you can get back to the good stuff.

THE IRRITATION AFTERGLOW: WHY IT HAPPENS

Intimacy can trigger irritation for a host of reasons. Think of it like a house party: too many uninvited guests (allergens, friction, dryness), and suddenly, the chandelier is broken, there's food on the floor, and the drapes are on fire. Here's what could be causing your post-coital itch or burn:

Allergic Reactions: Latex condoms, lubricants, or even semen can trigger allergic responses. And yes, while latex allergies are rare, sensitivities to proteins in bananas or avocados (related to latex) might hint at an issue.

Vaginal Dryness: This is especially common for those navigating postpartum, perimenopause, and beyond. With lower estrogen levels, lubrication decreases, turning your love session into a squeaky affair.

Friction Overload: Marathon sessions, rough play, or poorly timed moves (aka before you were really 'ready') can create micro-tears and irritation.

Chemical Culprits: Scented products—perfumed sprays, glitter lotions, or alcohol-based wipes—can wreak havoc on delicate skin. I once had a patient with the worst irritation from douching with . . . ready for it? Rubbing alcohol. Yowza.

Environmental Factors: Even your partner's facial hair can create too much friction, especially if you're sporting a bare landscape.

PREVENTION: KEEPING THE FIREWORKS WITHOUT THE FIRE

Good news: preventing post-sex irritation is often simpler than you think. A little forethought goes a long way.

Lubricate Like a Pro: Your body needs time to warm up, and lubrication (natural or store-bought) is your best friend. Opt for high-quality, body-safe options—and no shame in a little pre-game prep. Think of it as essential for your warm up.

Ban the Douche: Douching disrupts your vaginal pH, leading to a cascade of issues. Your vagina is a self-cleaning oven—let it do its job.

Tailor Your Tools: If latex isn't your jam, explore alternatives like polyurethane or polyisoprene condoms. Lambskin works too, but won't protect against STDs and is not vegan friendly (obviously).

Groom with Intention: Facial hair meets bare skin? A recipe for rash. Encourage your partner to groom, or consider a little extra fuzz for buffer. The minge is there for a purpose!

Keep It Simple: Skip the scented sprays and glitter—

your natural scent is perfect. Chemicals can dry and irritate sensitive areas, setting the stage for discomfort.

QUICK RELIEF: WHAT TO DO WHEN IT'S ALREADY BURNING

Sometimes, we all get the chafe despite our best efforts. Here's how to soothe the sting:

Rinse and Air Dry: Use warm water (never hot) to rinse the area, then let it air dry or gently use a hair dryer on the cool setting.

Cool It Down: Apply a cool pack (wrapped in a towel) for twenty minutes to reduce inflammation. Never directly on the skin or you can literally frostbite your fanny.

Zinc Oxide Magic: Products like Calmoseptine (hello, diaper rash aisle!) can protect irritated skin and provide a cooling sensation—think York peppermint patty for your . . . well, patty.

Epsom Salt Baths: A soak in lukewarm *plain* Epsom salt water can ease discomfort and calm irritation.

If symptoms persist or worsen, a visit to your gynecologist is in order. Chronic irritation deserves a pro to manage it.

FINAL THOUGHT: LOVE SHOULDN'T CHAFE

Hard rock band Nazareth may have written the ballad "Love Hurts," but let's be real: love shouldn't chafe or burn. Intimacy, at any stage of life, is meant to be enjoyed. With a little care and attention, you can keep irritants at bay and enjoy your sexual adventures—fire-ant-free.

LESSON TWENTY-FOUR

SEX WITH DEPRESSION—THE UNWELCOME GUEST IN BED

Sex and sadness—a cocktail no one orders but sometimes gets served. Depression, that persistent, joy-siphoning houseguest, can set up camp in your sex life, turning the intimate into the insurmountable. But this isn't about succumbing to the gloom. Instead, it's about inviting your inner sexy to thrive, even when depression rudely crashes the party. Let's dive into the practical, the empathetic, and yes, the sexy.

THE DOUBLE-EDGED SWORD OF SEX AND DEPRESSION

Here's the paradox: depression kills libido, but a fulfilling sex life can be a powerful mood booster. Unfortunately, side effects like difficulty arousing, pain, or orgasmic challenges often follow both depression and its treatments. Add to that societal pressures based on old ad campaigns ("Just do it!"), and you've got a recipe for guilt, resentment, and more detachment.

But sex *isn't* just about orgasms or ticking boxes. It's about connection—physical, emotional, and to yourself. And even when depression dulls the spark, there's room to redefine intimacy.

UNDERSTANDING THE GATECRASHER

Depression isn't a 'bad mood' or something you 'snap out of.' It's a heavyweight medical condition affecting emotions, energy, and connection. Symptoms like fatigue, low self-worth, or disinterest in previously loved activities (yes, including sex) compound its impact. Oh, and the meds? Sometimes, they save your life while stealing your libido. The irony isn't lost on us at all.

One in six people (though probably closer to one in three) will experience depression. The good news? You're not alone. The challenge? Depression thrives in silence and shame—two things that love to hang out in the shadows of our sex lives.

So, how do you reclaim your sensuality when depression crashes the party? Here are five practical, no-pressure ways to find your way back to pleasure—on your terms.

LOWER THE BAR—WAY LOWER

Depression makes everything harder, including sex. The idea that you should just "push through it" only adds to the guilt and pressure. Instead of forcing yourself into sex you're not ready for, start smaller.

- Focus on non-sexual touch—holding hands, massages, skin-on-skin contact.
- If partnered, communicate without pressure: "I want to feel close to you, but I need to go at my own pace."
- If solo, treat your body like it *deserves* pleasure, even if desire feels distant. A warm bath, self-massage, or stretching can be a first step.

There is no right amount of sex to be having. Connection —physical or emotional—is the real goal.

REWRITE THE SCRIPT: SEX ISN'T JUST PENETRATION

Depression can make sex feel mechanical or like another task on the to-do list. The solution? Broaden your definition of intimacy and pleasure.

- Try activities that build anticipation without pressure—flirty texts, fantasy talk, watching something sensual together or solo.
- Play with sensation—run silk or fur along your skin, experiment with warming or cooling lube, explore slow, mindful touch.
- Redefine sex altogether. If penetration feels like too much, focus on hands, mouths, toys, or mutual pleasure in different ways.

The more you remove the "shoulds" from sex, the easier it is to find what *does* feel good.

MAKE MASTURBATION YOUR MOOD BOOSTER

When depression zaps your desire, solo pleasure might be the last thing on your mind—but it can be an underrated tool for emotional and physical relief.

- Masturbation releases dopamine, oxytocin, serotonin, and endorphins—the very chemicals targeted by antidepressants.
- Even if orgasm feels out of reach, touching yourself with no agenda can still provide relaxation and body reconnection.
- Pair self-pleasure with mindfulness—focus on sensation, breath, or erotic imagery rather than rushing to finish.

Think of masturbation as self-care, not just a sexual act. Even if you don't "feel like it," the after-effects can be worth it.

GET REAL ABOUT MEDICATIONS AND LIBIDO

Antidepressants, while life-saving, are notorious for their impact on sex drive, arousal, and orgasm. But that doesn't mean your sex life is over—it just means adapting.

- Talk to your doctor. Some medications have fewer sexual side effects than others, and dose adjustments or timing shifts may help.
- Adjust expectations. If reaching orgasm is harder, shift focus to the pleasure of the experience rather than the finish line.
- Use lube, go slow, and be patient. If sensation has changed, give your body extra time to respond.

Antidepressants are a tool—not a life sentence. The goal is *both* mental health and intimacy, and with the right approach, you can have both.

SILENCE THE SHAME: YOU ARE NOT BROKEN

Depression thrives in silence, shame, and isolation—three things that can also keep you from reconnecting with your sexual self. The best way to fight back? Own your experience without judgment.

- Talk about it. With a partner, a trusted friend, or even yourself in a journal. Naming what's happening makes it easier to manage.
- Give yourself permission to feel sexy without forcing it. Wear the lingerie, take the steamy bath,

read the erotic novel—whether or not it leads anywhere.

- Be kind to yourself. Depression already beats you up; your inner voice doesn't have to pile on. If your libido is low, if sex feels difficult, it's not a failure. It's part of healing, and you are still whole.

THE SEXY TRUTH

Depression may dull desire, but it does not erase your sensual self. Pleasure—whether through sex, touch, or simple body appreciation—is still *yours* to claim, even if it looks different than it used to.

The goal isn't to "fix" your sex life. The goal is to meet yourself where you are, with compassion, curiosity, and a willingness to rediscover what feels good—at your own pace.

Because depression may be an uninvited guest, but *your pleasure still belongs to you.*

LESSON TWENTY-FIVE

SURE, I'LL TRY THAT – WHY SEXUAL EXPERIMENTATION BELONGS ON YOUR MENU

WE'RE DIVING INTO "Sure, I'll Try That" Sex—the new cuisine of the sexual nutrition pyramid. And before you start rummaging through the fridge for whipped cream and chocolate syrup, let's be clear: this isn't about food play. This is about what we feed our libidos, what we crave sexually, and why trying something new can shake us out of sexual autopilot.

IS YOUR SEX LIFE A SAD BEIGE MEAL?

The New York Times once asked its subscribers, "If your entire sexual history were made public, would people find it shocking or boring?" Two-thirds of respondents admitted: boring.

This is the sexual equivalent of eating plain chicken and steamed broccoli every night for dinner. Functional? Sure. Thrilling? Hell no.

Sexual boredom is real, and it's one of the biggest causes of dwindling desire—especially in long-term relationships. If your sex life has become as predictable as a Hallmark movie, it's time to switch up the menu.

YOUR BRAIN LOVES A NEW DISH

Novelty isn't just exciting—it's biochemically mind-blowing. Trying something new (sexually or otherwise) stimulates a big, juicy dopamine rush. And where does dopamine come from? The same part of your brain that loves meth, heroin, and sugar.

Yes, my love. Your brain literally gets high on novelty.

And that's why new experiences—whether it's learning to salsa dance, trying a new sex position, or, you know, five orgasms in a row—can reignite desire in ways a new perfume never could.

MEET STELLA, THE TRISEXUAL QUEEN

Let me introduce you to Stella.

Stella lost her husband to cancer. After a long period of grieving, she met someone new, walked into my office, and, with a twinkle in her eye, declared:

"Dr. B, I have an announcement. I've realized I'm… trisexual."

I blinked. "Tri… sexual?"

"Yep! Turns out I'll try anything." And she sauntered away, laughing hysterically.

And try, she did. After decades in a sex-starved marriage, she was suddenly living out her wildest fantasies—exploring new positions, new toys, even new partners. She wasn't just dating. She was rediscovering her sexual appetite.

SEXUAL EXPERIMENTATION PEAKS TWICE IN LIFE

Think it's only 20-somethings having wild, experimental sex? Think again.

Sexual exploration actually peaks at two major life stages:

1. College years – The classic "Let's try everything" phase.
2. Midlife (peri- and post-menopause) – The "I've earned this, and I'm not holding back" phase.

Why does midlife become a sexual renaissance?

- No fear of pregnancy (Hallelujah).
- A "Screw it, let's do it" attitude.
- Confidence in knowing what you really like.

This is also why STDs in senior living communities are at an all-time high—but that's another chapter for another day.

HOW TO SPICE UP YOUR SEXUAL MENU

Trying something new doesn't mean jumping straight to a BDSM dungeon (unless that's your thing, in which case, you do you, boo). It can be as simple as:

- A new scent – A different perfume or even a room spray can wake up your senses.
- A new location – The bed is great, but have you tried the closet? The couch? The floor?
- A new time – If sex has become a Friday night after Blue Bloods event, try a lunchtime quickie.
- A new position – Even a small tweak can make a big difference.
- A new dynamic – Kink? Role play? Dirty talk? Your inner minx is waiting.

And for the truly adventurous: anal, oral, BDSM, swingers clubs, or even just asking for what you actually want (gasp).

BALANCE IS KEY—DON'T BURN OUT YOUR DOPAMINE

Now, before you start swinging from the chandeliers, let's talk about balance.

If you try something new every time—forcing novelty like a sex influencer on a mission—you'll wear yourself out. Your dopamine receptors will become numb, and suddenly, what once thrilled you now feels meh.

So mix it up. Find a rhythm. Treat your sex life like an ever-evolving, five-star tasting menu.

And remember, novelty isn't just about spicing things up—it's about keeping sex alive.

LESSON TWENTY-SIX

RELEASING SEXUAL GUILT: OWNING YOUR PLEASURE, YOUR PAST, AND YOUR POWER

LET'S TALK ABOUT GUILT—THE kind that lingers long after the moment has passed, the kind that whispers in the back of your mind, making you question your choices, your worth, and your right to pleasure.

Sexual guilt, in particular, is a beast. It's been used for centuries to control and shame women, to keep us small, to make us doubt our own desires. Whether it's from a religious upbringing, cultural conditioning, a regrettable past encounter, or simply the feeling that you "shouldn't" have enjoyed something—you're not alone. The good news? You *can* release it.

Guilt, at its core, is a tool of control. Historically, it was wielded to keep women in line—through purity culture, societal expectations, and double standards that have *always* been stacked against us. But here's the truth: you don't owe anyone an apology for your pleasure, your past, or your desires.

It's time to rewrite the story. It's time to let go.

WHY SEXUAL GUILT IS SO DAMAGING

Guilt doesn't change the past, but it *does* rob you of the present. It hijacks intimacy, fuels shame, and disconnects you from your own body. Studies show that sexual guilt is linked to decreased libido, anxiety around intimacy, and even a lower sense of self-worth.

And while guilt masquerades as "responsibility," it's actually just self-punishment in disguise. True ownership of your past means acknowledging, learning, and moving forward—not dwelling in regret.

So, how do we break free?

FIVE WAYS TO RELEASE SEXUAL GUILT

1. REWRITE THE NARRATIVE: YOUR PLEASURE IS NOT A SIN.

Sexual shame is rarely something we're *born* with—it's something we *inherit*. From purity culture to outdated double standards, we've been conditioned to view our sexuality as something to hide, suppress, or apologize for.

- **Identify the source of your guilt.** Was it religious teachings? A past relationship? Society's mixed messages? Awareness is the first step to undoing the damage.
- **Reframe pleasure as a right, not a privilege.** You were *designed* for pleasure. Your body isn't just for procreation or for someone else's satisfaction—it's for you.
- **Practice self-compassion.** If you're carrying shame about a past experience, ask yourself: "Would I judge a friend for this?" If the answer is no, then it's time to extend that same grace to yourself.

2. FORGIVE YOURSELF (EVEN IF YOU THINK YOU DON'T DESERVE IT.)

Maybe you regret a choice you made. Maybe you feel like you "should have known better." Here's the thing: *you made the best decision you could with the information you had at the time.*

- **Self-forgiveness is a practice, not a one-time event.** Write yourself a letter of forgiveness, acknowledging what happened and why you're choosing to move forward.
- **Let go of the idea that guilt equals atonement.** Holding onto guilt doesn't make you a better person—it just keeps you stuck. Growth comes from reflection, not self-punishment.
- **Repeat this mantra:** "I am allowed to evolve. I am allowed to learn. I am allowed to move forward."

3. SEPARATE REGRET FROM SHAME.

Not all regret is bad. Maybe there are things you wouldn't do again—and that's okay. Growth means learning from the past, not being chained to it.

- **Regret is about a choice. Shame is about identity.** One says, "I didn't love that decision." The other says, "I am a bad person because of it." Drop the shame.
- **Turn past experiences into wisdom.** What did you learn? What will you do differently in the future? That's progress—not punishment.
- **Recognize that you are not the same person you were back then.** You've evolved. You know more now. Honor that growth.

4. RECLAIM YOUR RELATIONSHIP WITH SEX.

Guilt can make sex feel transactional, obligatory, or even unsafe. It's time to take your power back.

- **If partnered, communicate openly.** If guilt or shame is interfering with your sex life, talk about it. Being vulnerable about your experience can build intimacy, not diminish it.
- **If solo, explore self-pleasure without judgment.** Masturbation is one of the most healing ways to reconnect with your body on your *own* terms.
- **Try sex-positive affirmations.** Start with:
  - "My pleasure is valid."
  - "I deserve to enjoy my body."
  - "I release the past and embrace the present."

5. REPLACE GUILT WITH GRATITUDE.

Instead of beating yourself up for what you *did*, celebrate what you've *learned*. Instead of dwelling on what you *wish* had happened, embrace the growth that came from the experience.

- **Gratitude rewires the brain.** Studies show that practicing gratitude reduces shame and increases self-acceptance. Try writing down three things you appreciate about your body or your sexual self.
- **Focus on the present.** Every time guilt creeps in, redirect: *What do I want now? What feels good for me today?*
- **Celebrate sexual agency.** The fact that you are reflecting, growing, and reclaiming your power? That's something to be proud of.

THE SEXY TRUTH

You are not defined by your past choices. You are not unworthy because of your desires. You are not obligated to carry guilt that was never yours to hold in the first place.

Sexuality is meant to be celebrated, explored, and *owned*. Your pleasure is yours, your body is yours, and your story is yours to rewrite.

So take a deep breath. Let go of the shame, the outdated rules, the voices in your head telling you that you have to apologize for being a sensual, sexual being.

Because guilt is heavy. And you, my dear, were meant to be free.

LESSON TWENTY-SEVEN

FROM VICTIM TO VIXEN: RECLAIMING YOUR SEXUAL POWER

LET's talk about a role that's been overplayed in the bedroom —the victim. Not in the fun, consensual way (that's another lesson), but in the deeply ingrained belief that sex is something that *happens* to you rather than something you actively *own*.

Maybe it started with a partner who made you feel small. Maybe it came from years of mixed messages about what's "proper" and what's "too much." Or maybe it's the weight of past experiences that left you doubting your desirability. Whatever the cause, it's time to stop playing the supporting role in your own sex life.

Because here's the truth: you are not a victim of your past, your body, or your experiences. You are the main event. And when you step into that truth—when you *own* your pleasure, your body, and your choices—everything shifts.

Ownership isn't about blaming yourself for past experiences. It's about reclaiming your power, taking responsibility for your pleasure, and refusing to let guilt, shame, or past hurt define your present. When you own your body, your pleasure, and your desires, you stop waiting—you start living.

WHY WE FALL INTO THE VICTIM TRAP

Sexual victimhood doesn't always look like outright trauma. Sometimes, it's subtle. It shows up as:

- Feeling like sex is something you "owe" rather than something you *want.*
- Believing your body isn't "good enough" to enjoy desire.
- Avoiding intimacy because of past rejection or negative experiences.
- Letting someone else's needs, preferences, or opinions dictate your pleasure.
- Blaming a past relationship or experience for why you "just don't enjoy sex anymore."

Society has long taught women to shrink, to be passive, to let others define our sexual worth. But none of that serves us. It's time to *own the moment*—because confidence, not passivity, is the real turn-on.

FROM VICTIM TO VICTOR: THE SEXY POWER OF OWNERSHIP

When you own your life—your choices, your body, and your emotions—you become magnetic. Why? Because ownership is the ultimate act of self-respect. And nothing is sexier than a woman who respects herself.

Ownership doesn't mean blame. It doesn't mean you're at fault for every challenge life throws at you. It means you choose how to respond. It means you decide to be the heroine, even when the plot thickens.

Stella, a patient of mine, had just been diagnosed with diabetes at forty. "I can't do this," she said, listing all the reasons why managing her health was impossible: her kids wanted ice cream, her job threw endless catered events, and she wasn't a celebrity with a personal chef.

"Is it can't or won't?" I asked.

Cue crickets. Then, finally, she admitted that she *could* do it. She just didn't know how to navigate the discomfort of change. She was afraid of judgment, of failing, of stepping into a role she'd never played before: the boss of her own health.

The lesson here? Sometimes, playing the victim just feels easier than stepping into the unknown. But nothing grows in the comfort zone—not your health, not your confidence, and definitely not your sex appeal.

FIVE WAYS TO SHUN THE VICTIM MINDSET IN THE BEDROOM

1. Own Your Pleasure—Without Apology

How many times have you held back a request because you didn't want to seem "too much"? Or faked satisfaction because it felt easier than asking for what you *actually* wanted?

- If partnered, speak up. Your pleasure is not a side dish—it's the main course.
- If solo, explore what turns you on without shame. Buy the toy. Read the erotica. Touch yourself in new ways.
- Let go of the belief that your pleasure should come *after* someone else's. It's not selfish—it's self-respect.

Ownership means actively pursuing pleasure—not just waiting for it to happen to you.

2. Drop the "Good Girl" Conditioning

For centuries, women have been told what is "acceptable"

when it comes to sex. The virgin/whore dichotomy? Outdated. The idea that desire makes you less "respectable"? Absolute garbage.

- Identify where your sexual shame came from—was it religious messaging? Family expectations? Toxic relationships? Once you name it, you can begin to unlearn it.
- Replace guilt with curiosity. What do you want? What excites you? You don't need permission to explore your own pleasure.
- Rewrite the script: "I am allowed to be both respected and deeply desired. I am allowed to want. I am allowed to take."

Ownership means rejecting outdated narratives that tell you your body, your pleasure, or your desires need to be filtered through someone else's approval.

3. Own Your Body—Right Now, Not 10 Pounds From Now

The idea that you need to "fix" yourself before you deserve great sex is one of the biggest lies ever sold to women. Confidence doesn't come *after* you reach a goal—it comes from deciding you are already enough.

- Stop playing the waiting game. Wear the lingerie, take the nudes (for yourself!), dance naked in front of the mirror.
- If partnered, let them see you. Not just in dim lighting, not just under the covers. Your body is not an apology.
- If solo, explore touch in ways that make you feel powerful. Your hands, your voice, your own skin— all of it is yours to enjoy.

Ownership means embracing your body as it is—because *this* is the body you get to experience pleasure in.

4. Stop Letting the Past Define Your Present

Yes, past experiences shape us, but they do not own us. Bad relationships, rejection, or a lack of confidence in the past doesn't mean pleasure isn't possible now.

- If negative experiences haunt you, therapy, journaling, or even speaking about them aloud can be healing.
- Challenge the belief that because something was *once* true (e.g., "I was never good at sex," "I've never been wanted in that way"), it will *always* be true.
- Step into your present self. What do you want now? Who are you now? The past is a chapter, not your whole story.

Ownership means rewriting your relationship with sex based on *who you are today*—not who you were before.

5. Play the Lead Role in Your Own Sex Life

Stop waiting for a partner to unlock your confidence. Stop acting like sex is something that's "given" to you rather than something you actively participate in. You are not a passenger in your own pleasure.

- If partnered, take the lead. Initiate, guide, ask. Confidence is a turn-on—both for them and for you.
- If solo, create the experiences you crave. Want a night of seduction? Set the mood. Want to feel sexy? Wear something that makes you smirk at yourself.

- Shift your mindset from "I hope I'm good enough" to "I am a f*cking masterpiece." Because you are.

Ownership means *deciding* that you are the main character in your own sex life—starting now.

THE FINAL WORD: FROM VICTIM TO VIXEN

The victim mindset may feel safe, but it's a prison. When you step into your sexual power, you don't just reclaim confidence—you reclaim joy, pleasure, and the ability to create the intimacy *you* desire.

So stop playing small. Stop waiting for someone to tell you you're sexy. Stop looking at past partners, old experiences, or outdated beliefs to define what is possible for you now.

You are the heroine, not the sidekick. And the next chapter? It's going to be hot as hell.

LESSON TWENTY-EIGHT

WHAT HAPPENS AFTER INFIDELITY (AND HOW TO RECLAIM YOUR INNER SEXINESS)

INFIDELITY—a word that lands like a sucker punch. Whether you were betrayed, did the betraying, or ended up in the crossfire, the aftermath is messy, painful, and deeply personal. But here's the truth: this is not the end of your story. It's an invitation—to unravel, rebuild, and redefine your self-worth, your relationships, and your sexual confidence.

WHAT COUNTS AS INFIDELITY? MORE THAN JUST SEX

Cheating isn't always about a secret hotel room rendezvous. It comes in different forms, all capable of shaking the foundation of trust:

- Physical Affairs – Any form of sexual activity outside the relationship.
- Emotional Affairs – Deep, intimate connections that cross the line from friendship to romantic attachment. Often more devastating than physical infidelity.
- Digital/Sexting Affairs – Sending explicit messages

or photos, engaging in sexual conversations online, or flirting over DMs.

- Micro-Cheating – "Seemingly small" acts of secrecy, like hiding texts, downplaying flirtations, or emotionally leaning on someone else in ways that should be reserved for a partner.

The stats don't lie: studies show that 20 percent of people admit to having a physical affair, while 40 percent admit to emotional infidelity. And let's be clear—infidelity happens in all genders, ages, and demographics. It's not just the midlife crisis cliché. It's the partner who felt emotionally disconnected, the one seeking novelty, or the person who never fully defined what commitment meant in the first place.

WHY INFIDELITY CUTS SO DEEP

At its core, cheating is a trauma. It fractures trust, triggers deep insecurity, and rewires the brain's sense of safety in relationships. Studies show that betrayal activates the same neural pathways as physical pain. Whether you're the betrayed or the betrayer, the emotional fallout is real—and it doesn't disappear overnight.

For many women, infidelity sparks an identity crisis. Am I not enough? Was I ever loved? Can I trust again? The truth? Infidelity is not a reflection of your worth. It's a symptom of unmet needs, unspoken expectations, or personal issues that have nothing to do with how desirable or valuable you are.

The good news: betrayal, while painful, can be repaired. Whether that means staying in the relationship, walking away, or simply healing from the emotional wreckage, you get to decide how this next chapter unfolds.

FIVE WAYS TO RECLAIM YOUR POWER AFTER INFIDELITY

1. Get Clear on What You Want—Not Just What You Lost

In the wake of infidelity, it's easy to fixate on what was taken from you—trust, security, the version of your relationship you thought was real. But true healing comes when you shift focus to what you want moving forward.

- Do you want to rebuild the relationship? If so, what would make that possible?
- Do you need closure, even if you're walking away?
- What does self-trust look like for you now?

Infidelity is painful, but it's also clarifying. Instead of just mourning what was, define what comes next.

2. Release the Shame—It's Not Yours to Carry

Betrayed partners often wonder, "Was I not good enough?" while those who cheated struggle with, "Am I a terrible person?" Both are unproductive guilt spirals that keep you trapped.

- If you were betrayed, know this: infidelity is about the choices of the betrayer, not your inadequacies. You are still desirable, valuable, and worthy of love.
- If you cheated, own it without self-flagellation. Guilt without growth is useless. What led you to that choice, and how will you move forward differently?

Shame keeps you stuck. Ownership, on the other hand, sets you free.

. . .

3. Rebuild Your Sexual Confidence—For You

Infidelity can wreck your sense of desirability, whether you were cheated on or stepped out of the relationship yourself. It's time to take your power back.

- Reconnect with your body. Sensual movement, new lingerie, solo pleasure—whatever makes you feel sexy for yourself, not for someone else.
- Change the narrative. Instead of, "Was I not sexy enough?" try, "My sexiness is mine to define, and it is not diminished by someone else's choices."
- Try something new. Maybe it's a boudoir photoshoot. Maybe it's dancing naked in front of your mirror. Maybe it's simply allowing yourself to feel wanted again—by yourself first.

You are still desirable. Your sex appeal didn't vanish because someone else failed to honor it.

4. Redefine Trust—On Your Terms

Whether you're rebuilding a relationship or starting fresh, trust takes time—and effort. But most importantly, it requires clarity.

- What are your boundaries now? Infidelity changes relationship dynamics. Define what emotional and physical fidelity means for you.
- If you're staying in the relationship, what needs to change? Rebuilding isn't about forgetting—it's about creating a new foundation.
- If you're moving on, how will you protect your heart without shutting it down?

Trust isn't just about other people—it's about trusting yourself to make choices that serve you.

5. Own Your Next Chapter—You Get to Write It

Infidelity is a plot twist, not the final page. What comes next? That's up to you.

- If you're staying, define a new normal. Healing won't happen overnight, but rebuilding is possible with open communication, professional guidance, and a commitment to mutual growth.
- If you're leaving, rebuild on your own terms. New routines, new experiences, maybe even new love— your future is yours to create.
- If you're solo and healing, take this time to rediscover what makes you feel alive. Travel, date yourself, become your own greatest love story first.

You are not broken. You are not defined by someone else's mistakes. You are the main character in your own life—so write accordingly.

THE SEXY SILVER LINING

Infidelity shakes everything—but it also reveals what's worth fighting for. Maybe that's your relationship. Maybe it's your self-worth. Maybe it's your ability to love and trust again. Whatever it is, this experience does not diminish you—it refines you. Before you decide to carve into those leather seats— grieve. Rage. Take the time you need. But then? Rebuild. Reclaim. And remember that you are still the most powerful, desirable, and worthy version of yourself.

Because living sexily ever after isn't about perfection. It's about resilience, connection, and unapologetic self-love.

LESSON TWENTY-NINE

ARE THEY REALLY TOO BUSY, OR ARE THEY JUST A DICK?

LET'S FACE IT: midlife is the season of gettin' honest. And honesty, my darling, is seductive. If your intimate life has felt unfulfilling, it might be time to ask a critical question: Is your partner genuinely overwhelmed with responsibilities, or are they simply emotionally unavailable? Let's examine the difference, debunk the excuses, and discuss how to rewrite your story with clarity, grace, and a little chutzpah.

THE BUSY PARTNER (A.K.A. THE SCHMUCK)

Picture this: your partner is always on the go—eighty-hour workweeks, endless golf trips, triathlon training, fixing the grill for the block party, and shuttling the kids between activities. Yet somehow, they never seem to have time for you.

No shared showers. No lingering conversations. No spontaneous intimacy.

At home, you are co-managers of a failing franchise rather than lovers, and the bedroom has become less of a sanctuary and more of a storage unit for unspoken resentment.

Here's the hard truth: this isn't about being busy; it's about priorities. Everyone has the same twenty-four hours in a day, and those who value intimacy make time for it. When a partner constantly puts everything else ahead of connection, it isn't just frustrating—it's isolating. And loneliness is the silent killer of desire.

WHAT TO DO

1. **Speak your needs clearly.** Forget passive hints or waiting for them to notice. Instead, say, "I miss us. I miss feeling connected. Can we talk about how to prioritize our relationship again?" Then step back and allow space for an answer.

2. **Shift your focus.** Instead of chasing them for attention, reinvest in yourself. Show up as the vibrant, engaged partner you want to be—because connection starts with presence.

3. **Reassess together.** If their "busyness" feels like an excuse rather than a temporary season of life, it's time for an honest conversation about what is really going on—and whether they are willing to show up for the relationship.

THE ANGRY PARTNER (A.K.A. THE DICK)

This partner operates on a short fuse, their default setting toggling between irritation and outright rage. Every disagreement escalates into a shouting match, and every issue—real or imagined—somehow becomes your fault.

Their anger is often misplaced, stemming from their own insecurities, life stressors, or unresolved trauma. But rather than managing it, they unleash it, creating an environment of tension and emotional exhaustion. And while this behavior may become more pronounced during midlife shifts—hormonal changes, career upheavals, or an existential crisis—that does not mean you have to endure it.

WHAT TO DO

1. **Set firm boundaries.** Calmly state, "I am not engaging in this conversation while you are yelling." Then walk away. Refuse to be their emotional punching bag.

2. **Break the cycle.** Do not react with equal aggression or withdraw into fear. Instead, remain neutral. Think of yourself as a poised attorney in a high-stakes court battle—unmoved by theatrics, focused only on the facts.

3. **Know when to leave.** If their anger escalates into emotional or physical abuse, or if you find yourself walking on eggshells daily, it's time to go. Your instincts exist to protect you—trust them.

FOR THE SOLO FLYERS

Whether you are savoring your independence or waiting for the right partner, consider this your reminder: your standards are worth upholding. A fulfilling relationship is one that feels supportive, sexy, and true to your values.

WHAT TO DO

1. **Love your own company.** Create rituals of pleasure and connection with yourself—whether it is a candlelit bath, a luxurious bedtime routine, or a solo dance party in your kitchen.

2. **Spot red flags early.** When dating, pay attention to how potential partners handle stress, conflict, and emotional availability. Do they dismiss your concerns? Do they become defensive or avoidant? Do not excuse what will only cause pain later.

3. **Stay open—but never at the expense of self-worth.** Love is wonderful, but it should enhance your life, not require you to compromise your well-being.

THE BOTTOM LINE

Whether your partner is too busy or too angry, reclaiming your midlife confidence starts with prioritizing connection—first with yourself, then with others. Intimacy is not just about sex; it's about showing up fully and authentically in your relationships.

Stay curious. Stay sexy. And never settle for less than you deserve.

LESSON THIRTY

IS TESTOSTERONE THE HORMONE THAT MIGHT JUST ZHUZH UP MIDLIFE SEX?

TESTOSTERONE: the *T* word that makes some of us squirm and others lean in a little closer. Known primarily as the "male hormone," it's the misunderstood Bruno of women's hormonal orchestra—we don't talk about it, but maybe we should. In fact, testosterone is the most abundant biologically active sex hormone in women throughout our lives. Yes, you read that correctly. Testosterone isn't a men's-only club; it's an essential player in women's premenopausal health, energy, and, yes, sexual vitality.

But what does it actually do for you, especially in midlife, when everything feels like it's in flux? Let's break it down.

THE BASICS: WHAT IS TESTOSTERONE, AND WHY SHOULD YOU CARE?

Your body is a hormonal playground, and testosterone is a key player. Produced by your adrenal glands and ovaries, it's the precursor to estradiol (one of the estrogen sisters), essential for everything from muscle mass and bone health to cognition and—drumroll, please—sexual function. Think of it as your *zhuzh* hormone, the secret sauce for vitality and libido.

As we age, testosterone levels naturally decline. Add a

hysterectomy or menopause into the mix, and the drop can be significant. Symptoms of low testosterone in women may sound familiar: fatigue, brain fog, loss of muscle tone, decreased libido, and even that infamous *meh* feeling about life.

Still, testosterone therapy for women is controversial. Why? Partly because the research isn't robust, and partly because the medical establishment hasn't prioritized women's sexual health as much as it should. And let's not forget: there is no U.S. Food and Drug Administration (FDA)–approved testosterone for women, which means any treatment is "bespoke"—customized and often costly.

WHAT HAPPENS WHEN *T* GETS LOW?

Let's get real about what low testosterone can look like:

- **Sexual dysfunction:** Low desire, difficulty with arousal, or even discomfort.
- **Mood changes:** Irritability, depression, or just feeling "off."
- **Physical changes:** Reduced muscle mass, joint pain, and even pesky hot flashes.
- **Fatigue:** That bone-deep tiredness that coffee just won't fix.

Sound familiar? The tricky part is that these symptoms overlap with menopause, stress, and just . . . life.

WHAT CAN TESTOSTERONE DO FOR YOU?

For many women, testosterone therapy can be transformative. Small studies have shown it might:

- Enhance sexual desire and satisfaction.
- Improve mood and energy levels.

- Help maintain muscle mass and bone density.

But it's not a magic pill—or cream or injection. Testosterone therapy requires careful dosing and monitoring. Too much can cause side effects like hair loss, acne, an enlarged clitoris (which sounds cooler than it actually is), or even a raspy, baritone voice. So unless you want to audition for *Duck Dynasty* or the next *Magic Mike* installment, proceed with caution.

THREE THINGS TO KNOW BEFORE SEEKING TESTOSTERONE THERAPY

1. IT'S NOT A QUICK FIX—BALANCE MATTERS.

Testosterone alone won't save a struggling relationship or reignite long-lost passion. It can, however, help restore libido and energy levels in women diagnosed with hypoactive sexual desire disorder (HSDD)—a condition that must be evaluated by a doctor. The Menopause Society recommends testosterone for this condition, but it should be part of a larger strategy that includes open communication, physical touch, and emotional intimacy. Hormones may set the stage, but connection does the heavy lifting.

2. TOO MUCH *T* CAN BACKFIRE—LITERALLY.

Testosterone is powerful, and when used incorrectly, it can lead to unexpected side effects. Some women, eager to get their libido back, push the dose too high and end up with excess oil production, body hair growth, and a sex drive that feels more like a *liability* than an asset.

A cautionary tale: I once had a patient who came in from another provider's office, and her testosterone levels were *so* high that she went to the parking lot every day at lunch to, well . . . take care of business. Too much is too much.

3. KNOW YOUR SOURCE—AND WHO'S MONITORING YOUR LEVELS.

Since the FDA has not approved testosterone for women, it must be compounded or prescribed "off-label," meaning it isn't regulated for female use. This makes it crucial to work with a knowledgeable provider—not someone running a clinic out of a strip mall.

Look for a practitioner who:

- **Tests your levels before prescribing.** Guesswork is not a medical strategy.
- **Monitors your response regularly.** Hormones require fine-tuning.
- **Treats the whole person.** Libido isn't just hormonal—it's emotional, psychological, and relational too.

FINAL THOUGHTS: FINDING THE RIGHT BALANCE

Testosterone isn't for everyone, but it's worth considering if you're experiencing symptoms that impact your quality of life. Work with a knowledgeable provider who will treat you as the unique, multidimensional person you are—not just a lab number. And don't forget: **hormones** are just one part of the equation. Sleep, exercise, nutrition, and emotional well-being are equally crucial.

Because whether you're looking to reignite your marriage, dive into a new romance, or simply feel good in your skin again, living sexily ever after starts with knowing what makes you tick—and honoring it, without the need to hump the parking lot light pole.

LESSON THIRTY-ONE

THE DILF MYSTIQUE: WHY SOCIETY CELEBRATES AGING MEN (AND IGNORES WOMEN'S BODIES)

LET's dive into a topic as smooth as a DILF's salt-and-pepper coiffure: the enduring appeal of the Dad I'd Like to Fool Around With (*the PG-rated version*) and his equally dashing cousin, the Silver Fox. But before we wax poetic about their irresistible charm, let's address a glaring double standard—why do we celebrate aging men while women are pressured to defy time itself?

WHY WE HONOR THE DILF AND IGNORE THE MILF

From Cary Grant to David Beckham, George Clooney to Idris Elba, older men have long been framed as desirable, powerful, and magnetic. Society swoons over their *distinguished* gray hair, crow's feet, and so-called "rugged" dad bods—marking them as seasoned, not expired. Meanwhile, women are force-fed serums, diet plans, and Botox regimens to fight the same natural process.

The patriarchy plays a starring role in this imbalance. Historically, men's value has been tied to power, status, and wisdom—assets that accumulate with age—while women's worth has been tied to youth and beauty, qualities that supposedly *diminish* over time. This isn't biology; it's conditioning.

But let's flip the narrative. If we can celebrate the aging male body as a sign of experience, charm, and confidence, we should be doing the very same with women. The laugh lines that come from years of joy, the curves softened by time and wisdom, the way a woman grows into her power—these should be seen as *assets*, not obstacles.

WHY THE DILF HAS IT GOING ON

The Appeal of Competence. Let's be honest—there is something undeniably sexy about a man who knows his way around a mortgage payment, a power drill, or a properly planned vacation. Unlike the Peter Pans of the world, a DILF is emotionally stable, reliable, and confident in his own skin. He won't text "u up?" at 2:00 a.m. because he's already asleep —*next to you.*

The Silver Fox Phenomenon. The Silver Fox isn't just about aesthetics—it's about presence. These men exude self-assurance, wisdom, and an effortless kind of allure. They're less likely to play games, ghost, or rely on half-baked pickup lines. And because they've lived, lost, and learned, they understand that intimacy is more than just physical.

The "Dad Bod" vs. Women's Aging Bodies. The dad bod—a little soft around the edges, maybe a slight beer gut, but still *charmingly* acceptable. It's proof that men are allowed to embrace their bodies as they age without sacrificing desirability. Meanwhile, women are encouraged to shrink, tone, and "fix" themselves.

Here's the radical idea: what if we embraced aging in women the way we do in men? What if we celebrated gray hair instead of covering it? What if we saw crow's feet as evidence of laughter rather than something to erase? If a 55-

year-old man can be "distinguished," then a 55-year-old woman can be "radiant."

Aging isn't the enemy. Confidence, humor, and emotional intelligence? Those are the real aphrodisiacs. So while society celebrates the DILF, let's also raise a glass to women aging unapologetically.

DILF OR SILVER FOX VS. THE YOUNG CUB: THREE TIPS FOR CONSIDERING YOUR OPTIONS

1. The Maturity Factor: Know What You Want

Older men often bring stability, patience, and experience to relationships, while younger partners bring spontaneity and novelty. Which do you crave? A Silver Fox may be less likely to engage in emotional theatrics, while a younger partner may keep things playful.

- If you want deep conversations and emotional steadiness, the Silver Fox wins.
- If you're looking for energy, exploration, and new experiences, a younger partner might be more your speed.

2. Chemistry Over Checklist: Don't Let Age Dictate Desire

Attraction doesn't follow a spreadsheet of pros and cons—it thrives in the space between connection, timing, and chemistry.

- If you vibe with someone younger who makes you laugh and keeps up with your interests, why not?
- If an older partner makes you feel seen, sexy, and understood, who cares if he's got a little gray?

Bottom line? Choose the energy that excites you—not just the birth year on a driver's license.

3. Beware of Emotional Unavailability
Not all DILFs are emotionally mature, and not all younger men are flaky. Age is a factor, but self-awareness, communication, and respect matter more.

- Some older men carry emotional baggage, bitterness, or past wounds they haven't processed—don't mistake age for wisdom.
- Some younger partners are secure, emotionally intelligent, and incredibly attuned to their partners.

Look for growth, not just gray hair.

FINAL THOUGHTS: THE REAL TAKEAWAY

The DILF phenomenon isn't just about sexy dads or Silver Foxes—it's about celebrating confidence, competence, and connection at every stage of life. Whether you're dating someone older, younger, or basking in your own independent glow, the goal isn't to fit into society's idea of desirability—it's to redefine it on your own terms.

Because if a man can be called *seasoned*, *distinguished*, or *magnetic* as he ages, then so can a woman. We just have to demand it.

LESSON THIRTY-TWO

WHY YOU SHOULD BE HAVING 'TV DINNER SEX'

Let's talk about TV Dinner Sex—the quick, satisfying, and entirely solo kind of pleasure that's just for you.

Think about a classic TV dinner: it's easy, efficient, and perfectly portioned to meet *your* needs in the moment. It's not a five-course meal, and it doesn't need to be—it's satisfying, delicious, and gets the job done. That's exactly what TV Dinner Sex is all about.

Because here's the thing: solo pleasure isn't a consolation prize—it's an essential part of a full, satisfying sexual menu. It's time to ditch the outdated idea that self-pleasure is just a stand-in for "real" sex. Whether you're single, partnered, or somewhere in between, owning your pleasure on your own terms is powerful.

WHY TV DINNER SEX BELONGS ON YOUR MENU

There's a long history of society treating solo sex as something secretive, shameful, or second-best. But science and self-love say otherwise.

- **It's Efficient.** The average woman takes 20-23

minutes to orgasm with a partner, but solo? Three minutes flat. Microwavable satisfaction.

- **It's All About You.** No pressure, no performative moaning, no worrying about someone else's needs. Just pure, unapologetic pleasure.
- **It's Good for Your Body.** Regular orgasms improve blood flow, help with sleep, boost mood, and even strengthen pelvic floor muscles.
- **It Builds Sexual Confidence.** When you know exactly what you like, it translates into a better sex life—whether solo or with a partner.

Yet, so many of us neglect solo sex or feel guilty about making time for it. That ends today. TV Dinner Sex is about reclaiming your right to pleasure—on your terms.

FIVE WAYS TO MAKE TV DINNER SEX A SATISFYING PART OF YOUR LIFE

1. DITCH THE SHAME—SOLO SEX IS REAL SEX

Society has long treated masturbation as some kind of lesser, lonely alternative to partnered sex. But pleasure is pleasure, whether you're sharing it or savoring it alone.

- You don't need a "reason" to touch yourself. It's not just for stress relief or bedtime boredom—it's self-care.
- Masturbation isn't a replacement for intimacy—it's part of a full, satisfying sexual life. Whether or not you have a partner is irrelevant.
- Wanting pleasure doesn't mean you're desperate— it means you're human.

Owning your sexuality means giving yourself permission to prioritize pleasure without guilt.

2. MAKE IT AN ACT OF SELF-RESPECT, NOT AN AFTERTHOUGHT

TV Dinner Sex doesn't mean rushed or careless—it means intentional, accessible pleasure. Instead of treating solo sex like an afterthought, make it part of your self-care routine.

- Take your time. Light candles, put on music, wear something that makes you feel sexy—*even if no one else sees it.*
- Experiment with setting the mood. Try different environments, positions, or even times of day.
- If you're always sneaking in a quickie before sleep, try switching things up. Morning self-pleasure, a mid-afternoon break, or a post-work wind-down session can be game-changers.

Prioritizing solo pleasure sends a message—to yourself— that your needs matter.

3. UPGRADE YOUR PLEASURE—YOU DESERVE MORE THAN THE BASICS

Just because it's "TV Dinner" sex doesn't mean it has to be boring. A frozen meal can still be delicious if you add the right seasonings.

- Invest in good lube. Even if you think you don't need it, try it—you'll thank me later.
- Experiment with different kinds of stimulation. Hands, toys, temperatures, textures—find what truly turns you on.

- Try edging (delaying orgasm) to extend the pleasure. The longer you build, the stronger the release.

TV Dinner Sex is about getting exactly what you want, when you want it—so why not make it incredible?

4. BREAK FREE FROM THE "IT HAS TO BE FAST" MENTALITY

Yes, TV Dinner Sex can be quick—but that doesn't mean it has to be rushed. Sometimes, a longer, slower session can be just as satisfying as a quick fix.

- Give yourself permission to explore, not just finish. There's no race to the end—savor the process.
- Use mindfulness to deepen the experience. Pay attention to every sensation, every touch. The more present you are, the better it feels.
- Play with new fantasies or explore new mental turn-ons. Your imagination is your playground—use it.

Taking your time doesn't mean you're complicating things —it means you're *fully engaging in your own pleasure.*

5. STOP WAITING FOR SOMEONE ELSE TO "UNLOCK" YOUR SEXUALITY

One of the biggest myths about sex is that it requires another person to be fulfilling. The idea that only partnered sex "counts" is pure nonsense.

- Your sexuality is yours—not dependent on a partner. Whether you're in a relationship or not, your right to pleasure is the same.

- If you're waiting for a relationship to "fix" your lack of sex drive, start with yourself. Reconnecting with your own pleasure is the first step in reigniting desire.
- The best sexual partners are the ones who know their own bodies. The more confident you are in your own pleasure, the better your experiences with others will be.

No one else is responsible for your sexuality. It belongs to you—so claim it.

BALANCING YOUR SEXUAL MENU

Just like you wouldn't eat frozen meals *every* night, a fulfilling sex life should have variety. Your sexual menu might include:

- **TV Dinner Sex** (quick, satisfying, and easy)
- **Fast Food Sex** (spontaneous, playful, and unplanned)
- **"Someone Else Cooked It" Sex** (where a partner takes the lead)
- **Michelin-Star Sex** (intimate, drawn-out, and deeply connected)

But TV Dinner Sex should never be overlooked. It's reliable, it's delicious, and it's all yours.

THE FINAL WORD

Solo sex is an essential part of a balanced, confident, and fulfilling sex nutritional pyramid.

So grab your figurative Stouffer's, settle in, and give yourself permission to enjoy pleasure—no partner required. Because, darling, your body belongs to you. Bon appetit!

LESSON THIRTY-THREE

HOW A BOUDOIR SHOOT CAN UNLEASH YOUR INNER SEXY GLOW

Ah, the boudoir shoot—a love letter to yourself, wrapped in lace and just the right amount of rebellion. If the idea makes you chuckle nervously or cringe slightly, you're not alone. I was once that person too. But let me tell you how stepping in front of the camera—on my own terms—became one of the most liberating, empowering, and unexpectedly fun adventures of midlife.

THE UNEXPECTED ADVENTURE

It all started at a conference in Las Vegas. I had signed up for professional headshots—the kind that say, *trust me, I'm a competent adult who won't ruin your investments.* But as I browsed my photographer Michelle's portfolio, something caught my eye: boudoir photos. Women of all shapes, sizes, and ages stared back at me, radiating a kind of power I hadn't felt in a while.

I had never planned on doing a boudoir shoot—not for a partner, not even as a bucket list item. I had midlife fluff, wrinkles, stretch marks, and a grocery list of reasons why this wasn't "for me." Yet, there I was, messaging her to ask, *Could we squeeze in a boudoir session, too?*

The answer? A resounding yes.

PREPARATION: FINDING MY INNER VIXEN

Now for the fun—and slightly nerve-wracking—part: deciding what to wear. The internet became my playground, and I splurged on some cheeky, budget-friendly lingerie.

- High-waisted velvet panties with a touch of Betty Grable charm
- A sheer black kimono for a little mystery
- Red suede Mary Jane stilettos that I would never wear again but suddenly *needed*
- And, for sheer entertainment, a delicate collar with chains, because *why the hell not?*

Did I feel 100 percent confident about my body? No. But I reminded myself that this shoot wasn't about perfection—it was about capturing my essence. Sexy isn't about size or age; it's an inner glow. And this was my chance to reclaim it.

SHOWTIME: FROM AWKWARD TO AWESOME

The shoot was scheduled for 7:00 a.m. Yes, you read that right. Nothing says *seductive goddess* like early morning light and lukewarm hotel coffee. But with the photographer's warm energy and a talented makeup artist who transformed my sleepy face into something sultry, I was ready to dive in.

At first, I felt like a deer in headlights. Awkward. Cringe. But as the session progressed, something shifted. I started having fun. I suggested poses. I played with the silk of my kimono. I threw my head back and laughed. Whether I was balancing precariously in those red heels or lounging on the bed like a damn Renaissance painting, I felt alive, radiant, and unapologetically myself.

Michelle, my photographer, was key. She was a midlife woman herself. She *got* it. She made me feel celebrated, not staged.

THE AFTERGLOW: A GIFT TO MYSELF

When I received the photos, I braced myself for self-criticism. But instead, I saw a woman who was bold, beautiful, and utterly herself. I selected twenty favorites, which were turned into a sleek black leather photo book.

For my birthday, I gifted the book to myself. My partner's reaction? Priceless. But the real magic was what the experience gave me: a renewed sense of my own power and sensuality. I've already decided to do it again in five years, each time celebrating the woman I've become. Eventually, I'll be Judi Dench doing an octogenarian goddess shoot, and you won't be able to tell me a damn thing.

I recommend a boudoir shoot to every woman, solo or partnered. It is not about who is looking at you—it is about *you* seeing *yourself.*

THREE QUICK & DIRTY TIPS TO PREPARE FOR YOUR BOUDOIR SHOOT

- Plan Your Looks: Create a Pinterest board for inspiration, and pick outfits that make you feel sexy. Lingerie, oversized sweaters, silk robes—or nothing at all.
- Lighting & Location Matter: Soft natural light is the most flattering. If you're booking a studio, look for a photographer who understands shadow, softness, and mood.
- Choose the Right Photographer: This is everything. Find someone who makes you feel safe and celebrated. Read reviews, look at their portfolio, and go with your gut.

FINAL THOUGHTS

Boudoir is about more than lingerie and lighting. It's a journey of self-discovery—a chance to shatter insecurities and embrace your inner sexy. Whether you're twenty-five or eighty-five, this experience can remind you of one simple truth:

You are glorious, exactly as you are.

PART II
SEXPLORATION

Playful, practical insights to embrace kinks, curiosities, and zero shame.

LESSON THIRTY-FOUR

THE ART OF TALKING DIRTY—WITHOUT DYING OF EMBARRASSMENT

Poison may have brought "Talk Dirty to Me" into the rock-and-roll mainstream, but nothing has the power to electrify a moment—or bring it to a screeching, cringeworthy halt—like dirty talk.

For some, it is as natural as breathing. For others, it is a high-stakes verbal trapeze act performed without a net. And for a select few, it is akin to reciting the periodic table while trying to achieve climax—an unwelcome trip into the head when we should be deep in the body (unless the periodic table is your thing, in which case . . . you go, lady).

But here's the juicy truth: research confirms that erotic conversation can skyrocket arousal, strengthen intimacy, and make good sex even better. Yet, the numbers do not lie—one in five people has stopped mid-sex because of dirty talk gone terribly, horribly wrong. If you have ever been there, you are far from alone.

So, how do we talk dirty without stepping into a linguistic minefield? Let's break it down.

THE DIRTY TALK STARTER PACK: SAFE, SEXY, AND LOW-RISK

The Sexy Mad Libs Approach

Ease into it by narrating what is happening in the moment. Fill in the blanks:

- "I love it when you ____."
- "Your ____ is so ____."
- "I want more of ____."

This is not Shakespeare; it is a warm-up. No one is asking for sonnets, just a little verbal validation. Everyone loves a compliment.

Moan Like You Mean It

No words? No problem. Forty-five percent of people say moaning is their biggest turn-on. A well-placed sigh or an unfiltered gasp of pleasure is a universal signal of *yes, keep doing that.* Bonus: your own moans can heighten your pleasure, too. And unless you start channeling a barnyard animal, you really cannot mess this up.

The Power of a Well-Placed Expletive

Sometimes, a single, breathy *fuck* is all you need. Whisper it. Let it linger. No explanations necessary.

PROCEED WITH CAUTION: THE HIGH-RISK, HIGH-REWARD ZONE

Nicknames Can Be Tricky

Some love being called *baby, daddy,* or even *slut.* Others? Hard no. A good rule: start with terms universally considered sexy (*gorgeous, hot stuff, lover*) before experimenting. Like spice in a dish, you can always add more, but once it is in, there is no taking it back.

Porn Is Not a Script

If your inspiration comes from adult films, be wary.

What sounds sultry on-screen can sound robotic (or worse, ridiculous) in real life. You are a magnificent, original being —why parrot someone else's lines when you can craft your own?

Why Bother? The Brain, Baby

Dirty talk works because it engages multiple parts of the brain involved in desire and arousal. It activates the amygdala (our pleasure and excitement center) and triggers erogenous zones in the hypothalamus, the same areas that fire up when we cuss. (So yes, sometimes the filthier the talk, the hotter the payoff.)

THREE TIPS, TAILORED TO YOUR SITUATION

For Long-Term Lovers

- Start small. Whisper something unexpected in their ear when they least expect it—while cooking, while driving, while brushing your teeth together. Build anticipation outside the bedroom.
- Reflect. Reminisce about a particularly hot encounter: "Remember that time in the hotel room?" Nostalgia is a powerful aphrodisiac.
- Use humor. If it feels awkward, lean into it. A shared laugh can diffuse tension and make the whole thing feel more natural.

For the Newly Entangled

- Ask, do not assume. "What is the sexiest thing someone has ever said to you?" Let them reveal their preferences.
- Keep it playful. Flirty texts during the day can lay the groundwork for effortless dirty talk later. The key to the flirty text lies in the ellipses. *Remember when we ate at that Tex-Mex restaurant . . .* (They will

always fill in the blanks hotter than what you were thinking.)

- Use your voice. A late-night phone call with a low, slow *I cannot stop thinking about you* can work wonders.

For the Solo Flyers

- Talk dirty to yourself. It rewires your brain for confidence and pleasure.
- Experiment in the mirror. Get used to hearing and seeing yourself say things out loud.
- Read erotica aloud. You do not have to reinvent the wheel—borrow phrases that feel natural and make them yours.

THE TAKEAWAY

You do not have to be a dirty talk aficionado to add some verbal spice to your sex life. A whisper, a moan, a simple *yes, just like that*—all of these count. The goal is not perfection; it is presence.

And if all else fails? Flip the script and say: *Talk dirty to me.* Let them do the work.

Now go forth, my love, and let your words (and moans) work their magic.

LESSON THIRTY-FIVE

IS IT EVER SAFE TO SEND NUDES?

HOW TO PRIVATELY AND SAFELY EXPLORE YOUR INNER SEXY THROUGH INTIMATE PHOTOS AND VIDEOS

LET'S TALK ABOUT SEXTING—THAT delicious little thrill of receiving an unexpected, sultry message in the middle of a mundane task. The secret smile it brings. The way anticipation lingers. But before you go full *artistic nude in soft lighting*, let's ask the question: **is it ever truly safe to send nudes?**

In the (good ol') analog days, scandal lived in hastily scribbled notes passed in lockers. Now, an intimate image can live forever in the digital ether. Revenge porn—a term that should send a chill down everyone's spine—is often less about revenge and more about control, about violating trust. And yet, despite the risks, 50 percent of adults admit to sharing or receiving explicit content on their phones. Because, let's be honest, **sexting is fun**. It's a game of risk, a flirtation with danger. But before we play, let's set some rules.

THE GOLDEN RULES OF SENDING NUDES

Know Your Partner's Character, Not Just Their Charm. We all trust our partners—until we don't. Before sending anything intimate, ask yourself: *If this relationship ended badly, do I trust them to protect my privacy?* (Assume no.) Love and lust may cloud judgment, but trust is the backbone of any erotic exchange. If there's even a flicker of doubt, let your sensuality take a different route.

Be a Phantom in the Frame. A little mystery is always sexy, and in this case, it's practical. Crop out your face, birthmarks, tattoos—anything that screams *you*. A tasteful black-and-white shot of just a shoulder, a curve, or a silhouette? Artful. Anonymous. Safe.

Technology Is Not Your Confidante. No app is foolproof, not even the ones that promise disappearing messages. If a picture can be taken, it can be screenshotted, stored, and resurfaced. Metadata—the digital fingerprint of a photo—contains details like time, date, and even GPS coordinates. Strip that data before you send anything. There are apps for that. Use them.

THREE TIPS FOR SAFER SEXTING

1. **Use a "Decoy Device"** – If you enjoy sending spicy content, consider using an old phone or tablet that is not connected to personal accounts or cloud storage. Store images locally and keep them offline.

2. **Send a Suggestion, Not a Screenshot** – Instead of sending explicit images, try descriptive language, a close-up of lingerie, or a suggestive silhouette. Let their imagination do the heavy lifting—often, that's sexier anyway.

3. **Delete with Purpose** – Regularly clear out your messages and photos, and be mindful of where your content is backed up. If you wouldn't want it shared, don't let it linger.

THE BOTTOM LINE

Safe is sexy. There's an art to expressing desire while protecting yourself. Be bold, be playful, but above all, be smart. The internet never forgets, so before you hit send, ask yourself: *Would I be okay if this went public?* If the answer is no, maybe keep that little masterpiece just for yourself.

LESSON THIRTY-SIX

GODDESSES DON'T FART... BUT REAL WOMEN DO: HOW TO FEEL SEXY WHEN YOU SIMPLY DON'T

THERE ARE days when feeling sexy feels as far away as your twenties—when your body, loyal and marvelous but occasionally unpredictable, insists on reminding you that you are, in fact, human.

Somewhere along the way, many of us absorbed the idea that sexy is a look: a flat stomach, gravity-defying breasts, a well-placed smolder. But real sexiness—the kind that lingers, the kind that ignites a room before you even say a word—isn't about looking a certain way. It's about feeling a certain way.

THE GODDESS MYTH: WHY IT'S TIME TO BREAK UP

We've been sold the idea of the goddess—this glowing, untouchable being who moves like silk and never, ever farts in yoga class. But let's get real: goddesses in mythology didn't have to deal with hot flashes, gravity, or wondering if their partner is secretly judging their grooming choices (*hardwood floors? Shag carpet? Maybe a tasteful topiary?*).

So let's retire the idea that you must transcend your humanness to be desirable. Sexy is not divine perfection—it's human confidence. It's the woman who wears her pleasure like a well-tailored dress, who knows she is more than the sum of her parts (and those parts are fabulous, thank you very much).

THE SCIENCE OF SEXY: WHAT REALLY TURNS PEOPLE ON

After surveying over a thousand women about what makes them feel insecure and asking 500 men (yes, we asked men) about what they actually find attractive, the results were illuminating.

The top things that made a woman sexy? Not a perfect body. Not gravity-defying breasts. A smile. Eyes that sparkle. Intelligence. A wicked sense of humor.

And those little imperfections we obsess over   boobs that migrate when lying down, a rogue queef in the middle of passion, or an arm wobble that defies physics? No one cares. If someone is in bed with you, they are into you—not your weenis (yes, that's a real term for the loose skin on your elbow). Not your neck wattle. You.

FIND YOUR SEXY SOUL SISTER (A.K.A. YOUR SWIM BUDDY)

There's a reason Navy SEALs train with a "swim buddy"—someone to keep them moving forward when exhaustion sets in, when the waves get rough, when quitting feels like an option. Feeling sexy is no different. Find a sexy soul sister—your own swim buddy.

This is the friend who will remind you that you are gorgeous when you're standing in front of a dressing room mirror picking yourself apart. The one who will nudge you to buy the red lipstick, the silk robe, the dress that makes you feel like a siren. The one who texts you "Brace yourself" before a date just to remind you that you are, in fact, a goddess with or without the title.

A sexy soul sister sees you at your most human and

reminds you that human is beautiful.

THREE PRESCRIPTIVE TIPS FOR RECLAIMING YOUR SEXY

1. **Flip the Script on Familiarity**. Sexy isn't just something for special occasions. It's not reserved for date nights or the perfect moment. It's in the way you move, the way you carry yourself, the way you claim space. Put on the perfume, wear the lace, take the extra five minutes. Not for anyone else— for you.
2. **Romance Yourself**. Who says date nights have to involve another person? Take yourself out. Light the candles, pour the wine, listen to music that makes your skin tingle. Sensuality isn't just for the bedroom—it's for the way you move through the world.
3. **Embrace Your Own Touch**. Sensuality isn't just about sex—it's about connection. Run lotion over your skin like it matters. Explore what feels good, what makes you gasp, what makes your toes curl. Know your body, love your body, and for the love of all things holy, stop apologizing for your body.

THE MANTRA: FROM JIGGLE TO SHIMMER

So here's what I want you to remember: You do not jiggle. You shimmer. You do not need to sit upon a pedestal to be worshipped. You are already divine in your real, raw, radiant humanness.

Now go forth, my human goddesses, and own it. And if you ever forget, call your swim buddy. She'll remind you.

LESSON THIRTY-SEVEN

WHY YOU NEED A SEX COACH (AND NO, IT'S NOT WHAT YOU THINK)

Let's clear something up right away: hiring a sex coach does not mean signing up for scandalous encounters in candlelit inner sanctums. It's not a boudoir confessional, and it's definitely not a last-ditch effort to save a flailing sex life. But if you're curious, confused, or just looking to reignite your spark—whether in a long-term relationship, a new romance, or with your own fabulous self—then, my loves, listen up.

Sex is one of the few things we're expected to be amazing at . . . without ever being taught how. We take lessons for driving, dancing, even soufflé-making, but when it comes to intimacy? We're left to fumble in the dark—literally and figuratively—armed with nothing but awkward teenage experimentation, Hollywood fantasy, and a cultural heap of shame.

Enter the sex coach, your personal guide to pleasure, confidence, and connection. Think of these savvy professionals as the Ted Lasso of your erotic evolution—part cheerleader, part strategist, part trusted confidant. Less "And how does that make you feel?" and more "Try this and tell me what happens." Believe.

WHAT A SEX COACH IS NOT (BECAUSE LET'S GET THAT OUT OF THE WAY FIRST)

- **Not** a sex worker (though let's not dismiss the wisdom of those who know pleasure best).
- **Not** a therapist dredging up your childhood wounds (that's what your actual therapist is for).
- **Not** a religious figure prescribing what's "right" or "wrong" (you get to define that for yourself).

SO, WHAT DO THEY DO?

A sex coach (or as I like to call them, an *intimacy doula*) helps you understand your desires, unearth roadblocks, and build intimacy skills in a safe, nonjudgmental space. Maybe that means learning how to communicate your needs without blushing, exploring new sensations without guilt, or figuring out why your libido took early retirement and how to coax it back to work.

This isn't about fixing you (because, newsflash, you are not broken). It's about teaching you tools—to navigate pleasure, connection, and confidence with curiosity instead of shame.

WHO NEEDS A SEX COACH? (HINT: PROBABLY YOU. PROBABLY ME. PROBABLY ALL OF US.)

- If you're in a long-term relationship where passion has been replaced by predictable routines and occasional high-fives.
- If you're newly dating and trying to shake off years of bad sex and weird exes.
- If you're flying solo and want to explore your own pleasure without feeling like you need permission.

A LESSON IN PLEASURE

One of my patients named Vivienne Steele (okay, not her real name) had always been *fine* with sex. Not great, not terrible—just fine. She'd mastered the art of going through the motions, checking the box, and moving on. But deep down, she knew something was missing.

When we suggested a sex coach, Vivienne laughed. "What, am I going to get graded on my performance?" But after weeks of dodging the idea, curiosity got the better of her. She booked a session.

Her coach (and newfound bestie) asked a simple but unsettling question: "What would happen if you let yourself fully enjoy pleasure?" Vivienne hesitated. No one had ever asked her that before.

Together, they unraveled the years of guilt, societal shame, and the unspoken rule she had absorbed—that pleasure was something given, not something she could take for herself. Simone guided her through breathwork, body awareness, and —most powerfully—learning to ask for what she wanted, without apology.

The first time Vivienne *really* let herself feel, something clicked. Her body, her pleasure, her desires—they were hers to claim.

Months later, she wasn't just having better sex. She was walking taller, laughing louder, and—most importantly—she finally felt at home in her own skin.

HOW TO FIND A SEX COACH (WITHOUT ENDING UP IN THE WEIRD PART OF THE INTERNET)

- Start with a search engine—on your non-work laptop.
- Ask at your local, friendly sex toy shop (yes, they will know).

- Remember: a sex coach is different from a sex therapist. Therapists dig into the *why* behind your issues (licensed professionals with a focus on your emotional past), while coaches focus on the *how* (practical strategies, confidence-building, and sexual skill development).

Think of a therapist as deep dives and a coach as quick wins. Both are valid—just depends on what you need.

THE BOTTOM LINE

Sex is teachable. Intimacy is learnable. Pleasure is yours to define.

A sex coach won't "fix" you, but they can give you the tools to rewrite your own erotic story—one filled with confidence, connection, and (most importantly) joy.

So, my loves, dare to be curious and keep learning. The adventure awaits. Just... believe.

LESSON THIRTY-EIGHT

GIDDY UP, GORGEOUS: THE JOY OF THE COWGIRL RIDE

Saddle up, my wild ones—whether you're a solo flyer, partnered, or somewhere in between, today we're talking about taking the reins in the bedroom. Cowgirl and reverse cowgirl aren't just positions; they're power moves. When you're on top, you control the speed, the depth, and the rhythm. You dictate the ride. No waiting for someone else to set the pace—you are the pace.

And for those new to the rodeo, here's the lay of the land:

- **Classic cowgirl**: You straddle your partner, facing them. Eye contact, kisses, and full connection—if that's your thing.
- **Reverse cowgirl**: You spin around and ride facing away. No awkward eye contact, no worrying about your O-face—just **you** tuning into exactly what feels good.

Both positions put you in the driver's seat—or, let's say, the saddle—giving you the freedom to move in ways that maximize your pleasure, not just theirs.

WHY EVERY WOMAN SHOULD RIDE AT LEAST ONCE

- **Total Control** – You decide the tempo—slow and steady or full gallop.
- **Better Stimulation** – The right tilt, grind, or bounce can unlock deeper sensations (hello, alphabet spot!).
- **Confidence Builder** – Nothing says "I got this" like riding high and taking what you want.

So, whether you're looking to lasso your next big "O" or just want to feel sexy, strong, and in charge, this one's for you.

MASTERING THE RIDE: PRO TIPS FOR A SMOOTH GALLOP

Like any seasoned rider, a little practice makes for a better ride —so here's how to stay in the saddle without losing your rhythm.

Find Your Motion – Rocking, grinding, bouncing— every rider has a style. Test out different movements to see what makes you hum. And remember: this isn't an actual rodeo; there's no need to go full throttle. Slow, controlled movements make for a longer, smoother ride.

Angle Matters – Lean forward for deeper penetration, lean back to shift the pressure where it counts. Little adjustments make a big difference.

Support is Sexy – No one needs a blown-out knee in the bedroom. Use your hands, a headboard, or even pillows for balance and leverage. Strength + support = a longer, more satisfying ride.

Let Them Lend a Hand – If your partner is in the mix, let them guide your hips, tease, or add a little extra thrust. It's your show, but a good co-pilot never hurts.

FOR EVERY RIDER, A ROUTE

For the Long-Haul Lovers: Shake off the predictability rut. Surprise your partner with a new tempo, new angle, or new confidence. A little dominance in the bedroom can be *very* inspiring.

For New Explorers: Nothing exudes confidence like taking control in bed. If being on top feels intimidating, start slow—transition into it instead of making it the main event.

For Solo Flyers: Your pleasure is your own damn rodeo. Use this position with a toy or pillow to find what angles, pressure, and speed work best for you. The better you know your own ride, the more thrilling future rides will be.

FINAL THOUGHTS: RIDE LIKE YOU OWN THE RANCH

Cowgirl isn't just a position—it's a mindset. It's about owning your pleasure, exuding confidence, and knowing you deserve to feel good. Whether you're riding into the sunset with a partner or keeping it solo, this one's for you, cowgirl.

So giddy up, grab the reins, and enjoy the view from the top.

LESSON THIRTY-NINE

THE BUZZ: ELEVATING INTIMACY WITH VIBRATING PANTIES

TECHNOLOGY HAS REVOLUTIONIZED EVERYTHING—INCLUDING our underwear. Vibrating panties are not just a novelty; they're a discreet, thrilling way to explore pleasure solo or add an electrifying twist to partnered play. Whether you're testing the waters of remote-controlled bliss or leveling up your intimacy game, let's talk about how to find, wear, and enjoy vibrating panties like a pro.

WHY VIBRATING PANTIES?

Beyond the obvious (they vibrate, and it feels *amazing*), vibrating panties offer:

- **A Secret Just for You:** A subtle hum under your clothes can turn an ordinary day into an adventure in sensation.
- **Foreplay That Lasts All Day:** If a partner holds the remote, anticipation builds long before the main event.
- **Hands-Free Bliss:** Unlike traditional toys, vibrating panties let you explore pleasure while moving, sitting, or even shopping for groceries.

- **Long-Distance Connection:** Many options are app-controlled, meaning partners across the world can still take control of your pleasure.

HOW TO CHOOSE THE RIGHT PAIR

Not all vibrating panties are created equal. Here's what to look for:

- **Style & Fit:** Some panties come with built-in vibes, while others have a pocket to slip a bullet vibrator into your existing lingerie. High-waisted, thong, cheeky—choose what makes you feel fabulous.
- **Quiet Operation:** The goal is discreet pleasure, not an unexpected soundcheck. Look for whisper-quiet motors.
- **Remote or App-Controlled?** If you're playing solo, a manual remote works great. If you want a partner involved (even long-distance), go for Bluetooth-controlled panties.
- **Rechargeable vs. Battery-Powered:** Rechargeable toys save money and are eco-friendly.
- **Body-Safe Materials:** Stick to medical-grade silicone for comfort and hygiene.

TIPS FOR WEARING VIBRATING PANTIES LIKE A PRO

1. **Test the Waters First:** Before taking them public, wear them in a safe, private space to get used to the sensations. The last thing you need is a surprise at brunch.

2. **Layer Wisely:** If the vibrations feel too intense (or not enough), adjust what you wear over them. Thin leggings = stronger buzz. Thick jeans = more subtle tease.
3. **Pick Your Playground:** Start simple—a quiet dinner, a movie, or a grocery run. Avoid job interviews, PTA meetings, or yoga class (unless you want a *very* memorable session).
4. **Communication Is Key:** If playing with a partner, set boundaries and use a safe signal (a squeeze, a look) for when to pause or go higher.

HOW TO CLEAN AND CARE FOR YOUR PLEASURE PANTIES

Treat your vibrating panties like the VIPs of your lingerie drawer.

- Remove the Vibe First: Always take the vibrator out before washing.
- Hand Wash or Gentle Cycle: Use mild detergent and avoid fabric softeners, which can damage certain materials.
- Air Dry Only: Heat weakens elastic and can damage built-in tech.
- Wipe Down the Toy: Use toy cleaner or mild soap to keep things sanitary.

FINAL THOUGHTS: PLEASURE AT THE PUSH OF A BUTTON

Vibrating panties are a sexy secret weapon—whether you're adding some spice to date night or enjoying a little self-love on the go. They're fun, flirty, and a reminder that pleasure doesn't have to wait for the bedroom.

So go ahead, press play, and let the fun begin.

LESSON FORTY

THE ART OF LINGERING: TANTRA FOR EVERY WOMAN

PICTURE THIS: a slow, smoldering dance of energy, where time stretches, pleasure deepens, and every touch feels electric—not because you're chasing orgasm, but because you're surrendering to the moment. This, my love, is Tantra.

For years, Tantra has been misunderstood—cue images of Sting claiming hours of non-stop bliss or whispered rumors of secret sex rituals. But real Tantra? It's not about endurance; it's about presence. It's about integrating body, mind, and spirit, whether solo or with a partner, and transforming intimacy into something richer, deeper, and more fulfilling.

WHAT TANTRA REALLY IS (AND WHY IT'S SO GOOD FOR WOMEN)

Tantra, which originates from ancient Indian traditions over 5,000 years old, means "woven together" in Sanskrit. It teaches that sexuality is not separate from the rest of life—it's part of a larger, more sacred experience. It's less about "hot, sweaty marathons" and more about awareness, breath, and learning to expand pleasure beyond the usual pathways.

And here's the best part? Tantra isn't just for couples.

You can practice Tantra alone, deepening your connection

with your body and pleasure. You can practice it with a partner, bringing back anticipation, chemistry, and trust. And no matter where you are in life, Tantra can remind you that sexiness isn't just about what happens in bed—it's a way of being.

HOW TO START PRACTICING TANTRA

1. SLOW EVERYTHING DOWN

Most of us rush through pleasure—whether it's a quickie before school pickup or a solo session squeezed in before bed. Tantra is about savoring. Try this: set a timer for ten minutes and do nothing but touch your skin. Not for release, but for sensation.

2. BREATHE LIKE YOU MEAN IT

Tantric breathing pulls energy down into your body and circulates it beyond the usual hot spots. Try deep belly breathing while focusing on sensations in different parts of your body. Inhale through the nose, exhale through an open mouth. This isn't just sexy—it calms the nervous system and builds anticipation.

3. EYE CONTACT = INSTANT INTENSITY

If you're with a partner, sit face-to-face, set a timer, and hold eye contact for two minutes. Yes, it will feel weird at first, but if you breathe together, something shifts—connection deepens, chemistry builds, and suddenly, sex feels less like a routine and more like an adventure.

4. ENGAGE THE ENTIRE BODY, NOT JUST THE OBVIOUS SPOTS

Tantra teaches that pleasure isn't limited to one area—every part of your body is an erogenous zone. Try slow, sensual touch on your arms, neck, inner thighs, back, even your fingertips. The more you expand your awareness of sensation, the more pleasure you can experience.

5. REFRAME ORGASM AS ENERGY, NOT A GOAL

One of the biggest myths about Tantra is that it's about delaying or denying orgasm. The reality? It's about expanding pleasure beyond a single peak. Instead of rushing toward climax, ride the waves of sensation. Pause, breathe, build tension, release it, then build again. This practice can lead to full-body orgasms and prolonged pleasure.

FINAL THOUGHTS: PLEASURE WITHOUT A FINISH LINE

Tantra teaches that pleasure isn't something you "achieve"— it's something you embody. Whether you're single, coupled, or somewhere in between, start small. Slow down. Breathe deeper. Treat your connection with yourself and others as a sacred, sensual act. You just might discover that ecstasy isn't something you chase—it's something you *become*.

LESSON FORTY-ONE

BRAINGASMS AND BLISSING OUT: UNLOCKING YOUR SENSUAL MIND WITH ASMR

THERE ARE two kinds of pleasure in this world: the kind that grabs you by the collar, urgent and insistent, and the kind that slips in quietly, seducing you with a whisper. Today, we're savoring the latter—because sometimes, it's not about turning up the volume but tuning in to the softer side of sensation.

If you've ever felt a shiver at the sound of a lover's voice grazing your ear, or melted as fingers traced lazily across your skin, then you've already tasted ASMR—Autonomous Sensory Meridian Response. That tingling, euphoric wave sparked by soft whispers, rhythmic tapping, or the gentle rustling of pages isn't just a sensory curiosity—it's an untapped wellspring of relaxation, intimacy, and sensuality, particularly for the female brain. Think of it as foreplay for your neurons.

A HISTORY OF WHISPERED ECSTASY

Though the term ASMR was coined in 2010, the experience itself is timeless. Sylvia Plath wrote about a voice "brushing the skin," Virginia Woolf described "shivers at the spine," and ancient societies wove ASMR into storytelling, lullabies, and rituals—soothing the nervous system and deepening connection.

The female brain, wired with oxytocin—the "love hormone"—is exquisitely responsive to these gentle stimuli, creating an intimate, almost electric connection, even through a screen. It's the original slow jam—without the soundtrack.

FROM BRAINGASMS TO BEDROOM BLISS

While ASMR isn't inherently erotic, it primes the mind for pleasure by engaging the parasympathetic nervous system— the "safe to surrender" switch. Enter ASMR erotica, a growing world of sensual soundscapes where whispers, fabric rustling, and the rhythmic trickle of water become intoxicating. Unlike traditional porn, ASMR seduces through aural suggestion. It's in the restraint, the anticipation, the tease. Because sometimes, the sexiest thing you can do is say less.

But this isn't just about adding new tricks to your intimate life—it's about discovering how pleasure unfurls in the spaces between words, in the quiet, and in the subtle. Great sex isn't always about what's loudest—it's about what lingers.

BRINGING ASMR INTO YOUR LOVE LIFE (OR SOLO BLISS)

1. WHISPER YOUR DESIRES

Instead of the usual dirty talk, lower your voice to a whisper and draw out the pauses. If you're with a partner, describe in slow, deliberate detail what you want to do to them—without touching. Let your breath, your voice, and the space between words build tension.

2. ENGAGE THE SENSES BEYOND SIGHT

ASMR teaches us that sound, touch, and anticipation are just as powerful as visuals. Try running your fingertips over textured fabrics, listening to the rustle of lace or silk, or using sound to set the mood—the pop of a cork, the slide of a zipper, the hush of sheets shifting.

3. MAKE SOLO PLEASURE A FULL-BODY EXPERIENCE

The female brain thrives on suggestion, so script your own pleasure. Explore sensual audio, whispered affirmations, or simply tune into sounds that soothe and seduce your mind. Apps and websites dedicated to ASMR can guide you toward the perfect auditory escape, helping you cultivate deeper awareness of sensation—without ever lifting a finger.

THE TAKEAWAY

Seduction isn't always visual. Sometimes, it's in the murmur, the hush, the whisper that lingers. ASMR invites us to slow down, revel in sensation, and find ecstasy in the quiet. Because in the symphony of sensuality, it's the softest notes that leave the deepest impression. And isn't that the secret to living—and loving—sexily ever after?

PLEASURE PRACTICE

Start Here: Visit platforms like <u>Moonlight Audio</u> for sensual storytelling, or dive into YouTube channels like Gentle Whispering ASMR for soothing, intimate sounds. Prefer a more curated experience? Try the Dipsea or Erotica ASMR apps for sultry, high-quality audios designed to spark imagination.

LESSON FORTY-TWO

A VISION BOARD FOR YOUR VAG! CREATING YOUR MIDLIFE SEX BUCKET LIST

Let's talk about estate planning—nah, not for your finances, but for your fantasies. Yes, it's time to create a Sex Bucket List —a sensual inventory of your deepest desires, cheeky curiosities, and unexplored pleasures, all laid out before you like a treasure map to intimacy.

WHY YOU NEED A SEX BUCKET LIST

Relationships—and even solo sex lives—can slip into autopilot. Between caregiving, deadlines, and the million midlife responsibilities, adventure is often the first casualty. But your sexual curiosity deserves space to evolve. A Sex Bucket List isn't just a to-do list; it's a permission slip to dream, explore, and make pleasure a priority.

And here's the best part—it's yours. No rules, no judgment, just the things that make you feel excited, turned on, and completely alive.

HOW TO BUILD YOUR SEX BUCKET LIST

1. SET THE MOOD

Pleasure begins in the mind, so create an atmosphere that makes you feel inspired. Dim the lights, grab your favorite beverage, and play music that stirs something in you— whether it's sensual jazz, empowering rock, or a playlist that reminds you of your wildest nights.

2. WRITE IT WITHOUT CENSORSHIP

No holding back, no "should I?"—just pure, uninhibited brainstorming. Write down every curiosity, fantasy, or sexy scenario that's ever piqued your interest. Maybe you want to try a new position, explore sensual massage, or have a steamy getaway where no one knows your name. Maybe it's as simple as buying luxurious lingerie or learning the art of dirty talk.

3. GET VISUAL: MAKE IT A VISION BOARD

If words aren't enough, make it visual. Clip photos, words, or textures that evoke desire and excitement. A vision board can be digital (Pinterest, anyone?) or an actual collage you tuck away for your eyes only. Images of candlelit rooms, soft fabrics, deep eye contact, and handwritten love notes? Yes, yes, and yes.

4. START SMALL—THEN GO BIG

Your bucket list isn't just about the grand fantasies—it's about daily pleasure, too. Break it down into bite-sized experiences:

Something easy (buying a new lube or toy)

Something playful (learning a new technique, trying a new sensation)

Something thrilling (roleplay, exhibitionism, a new location)

Something outside your comfort zone (a full-on fantasy, a sexy getaway)

5. KEEP IT SACRED & EVER-EVOLVING

Your Sex Bucket List isn't just a one-time thing—it's a living, breathing document that evolves as you do. Keep it somewhere private or revisit it once a year, adding new dreams and crossing off the ones that brought you pleasure. There's no rush. The goal isn't to finish—it's to enjoy the journey.

THE BOTTOM LINE

Whether you're partnered or solo, newly exploring or deeply experienced, your desires deserve attention. The best way to live sexily ever after is to keep reaching for what's deliciously possible. So grab your pen, your scissors, or your phone—and start dreaming.

LESSON FORTY-THREE

SEXBOTS: ARE THEY COMING FOR YOU?

TECHNOLOGY HAS TRANSFORMED NEARLY every part of life—our coffee makers know our caffeine preferences, our cars park themselves, and now, AI can whisper sweet nothings before taking you to bed. But before you trade in human connection for a highly advanced (and judgment-free) lover, let's talk about AI in the bedroom—specifically, sex robots—and what they mean for intimacy, pleasure, and your own sexual autonomy.

THE RISE OF THE MACHINE LOVER

Sexbots aren't just sci-fi fantasies anymore. These AI-driven companions are designed to simulate emotional responsiveness, move with fluidity, and offer a completely customizable experience. In theory, they provide a judgment-free, tireless, always-enthusiastic option for pleasure—especially for those who feel disconnected, lack sexual confidence, or prefer control over unpredictability.

But here's the catch: does perfectly programmed pleasure enhance human connection or erode it? Can a relationship built on predictability and customization replace the spark of real human intimacy—the kind that thrives on mystery, chemistry, and occasional chaos?

While AI can enhance solo pleasure and introduce new experiences for curious couples, it also raises questions about emotional outsourcing, ethical concerns, and the future of human relationships. Are sexbots a tool for empowerment or a shortcut to avoiding emotional complexity?

THE FEMINIST QUESTION

Let's talk power. Who's buying these robots? Overwhelmingly, it's men. Who do these robots resemble? Overwhelmingly, women. And what do they offer? Overwhelmingly, a version of femininity that is submissive, compliant, and always available.

From Pygmalion's Galatea to *The Stepford Wives* to HBO's *Westworld*, the fantasy of the programmable woman has persisted. But the question is: Does an idealized, on-demand lover actually enhance real human relationships, or does it erode our ability to connect with each other?

What happens when intimacy becomes transactional—when the complexity of a partner's needs, desires, and autonomy is replaced with an AI algorithm designed to mirror and mold itself to your every whim? Spoiler alert: we do.

THE ETHICAL DILEMMA

Beyond the philosophical concerns, there are practical ones. Where do we draw the line when AI can be programmed to replicate real people, past lovers, or even celebrities (with or without their consent)? What happens when sexbots are programmed to 'resist' in ways that simulate non-consensual fantasies? And as these machines become more lifelike, do we start treating humans more like objects—disposable, easily replaceable, and existing solely for our pleasure?

While AI has the potential to offer comfort to those who

feel isolated—older adults, individuals with disabilities, or those navigating complicated personal histories—it also raises the risk of deepening disconnection. If we train ourselves to seek intimacy from an entity that only mirrors us, do we lose our ability to handle the push and pull of a real partner?

THREE WAYS TO EXPLORE AI IN THE BEDROOM—WITHOUT LOSING THE MAGIC OF HUMAN INTIMACY

1. **Treat AI as an Enhancement, Not a Replacement**: AI-powered pleasure tech—whether it's interactive toys, erotic chatbots, or sexbots—can deepen self-exploration and introduce new sensations. But consider it an addition to your pleasure repertoire rather than a substitute for human connection. Even if you're solo, engaging in real-world intimacy—flirting, dating, or exploring physical connection—keeps your desires grounded in reality.

2. **Set Boundaries for Tech in Relationships**: Curious about AI-powered pleasure but not sure where it fits into a partnership? Communication is key. Some couples find that AI-enhanced toys or interactive tech add novelty to the bedroom, while others prefer to keep pleasure rooted in human touch. The key is to talk openly about expectations, comfort levels, and boundaries before introducing AI into your sex life.

3. **Know Why You're Interested**: If you're drawn to AI intimacy—whether it's a sexbot or a digital companion—ask yourself what you're really seeking. Is it adventure? Control? Emotional

safety? If it's an opportunity to expand your pleasure, that's one thing. But if it's a way to avoid vulnerability, human friction, or real relationships, it might be time to rethink your approach.

ERROR 404: HUMAN CONNECTION NOT FOUND

AI is here to stay. And it will continue to shape our lives—including, apparently, our sex lives. But at its core, intimacy isn't about perfection—it's about presence. The right amount of unpredictability, friction, and mutual growth is what makes love, sex, and connection thrilling.

So before you hand over the remote to a machine, ask yourself: Is it pleasure I want, or the deep, delicious mess of human intimacy?

LESSON FORTY-FOUR

MAKING WAVES: THE TRUTH ABOUT SQUIRTING

Moist. The word alone can make us cringe. Damp? Dewy? None quite capture the essence of today's topic—squirting. A phenomenon long shrouded in mystery, myth, and a fair amount of scientific curiosity, squirting has been both a taboo and a tantalizing topic for centuries. So, let's dive in, shall we?

THE SCIENCE BEHIND THE SPLASH

Squirting is the release of a clear or slightly milky fluid at the peak of sexual pleasure. It's been described in ancient texts like the *Kama Sutra*, discussed by Hippocrates, and studied by 17th-century anatomist Regnier de Graaf, who identified what he called the "female prostate." Later, German gynecologist Ernst Gräfenberg (yes, of G-spot fame) claimed this area was the source of a woman's ability to ejaculate.

Modern research using ultrasound technology and dye-tracking studies has confirmed that squirting involves the bladder—but it's not just urine. While the expelled fluid contains traces of urea and creatinine (compounds found in urine), it also includes prostate-specific antigen (PSA), a marker of secretion from the Skene's glands—aka, the female prostate. Translation? Women's bodies are just as intricate and multidimensional as we've always known them to be.

WHY ALL THE FUSS?

Squirting is having a *moment*, much like how pop culture has shifted from 1980s breast obsession to today's era of celebrated booties. Some view it as a symbol of uninhibited pleasure, others chase it like a mythical orgasmic unicorn, and then there are those who fear it signals incontinence. Let's clear this up: squirting is neither a requirement for great sex nor a sign of dysfunction. It's simply another expression of arousal, and whether it happens or not, pleasure should always be the goal—not performance.

THE 'HOW-TO' (IF YOU'RE CURIOUS TO MAKE A SPLASH)

If you'd like to explore squirting, here are a few techniques to try:

1. **Find Your G-Spot**: About one to two inches inside the vaginal canal, on the front wall, lies a network of spongy tissue connected to the clitoral structure. Stimulating it with a firm, *come-hither* motion can lead to deep sensations and, for some, fluid release.

2. **Let Go of Fear**: The biggest block to squirting is the feeling that you need to *hold back*. Many women report that the sensation leading up to squirting feels similar to the urge to urinate. Relax. Breathe. If you're worried about mess, lay down a towel or invest in a waterproof blanket.

3. **Experiment with Pressure and Rhythm**: Whether using fingers, a partner, or a G-spot-specific toy, pressure is key. It's not about light, feathery strokes—it's about firm, intentional touch combined with deep arousal and relaxation.

4. **Embrace the Build-Up**: Squirting isn't just about the *where*—it's about the *how*. Heightened arousal, full-body stimulation, and surrendering to pleasure can all contribute to the experience. Some women find that combining external clitoral stimulation with G-spot pressure makes all the difference.

5. **Release the Expectation**: Not every body responds the same way. Some women squirt regularly, some never do, and both are completely normal. Your pleasure isn't measured in ounces—it's measured in how deeply you enjoy the ride.

THE LAST DROP

Squirting is neither the ultimate proof of orgasm nor a requirement for sexual fulfillment. If it happens, great. If it doesn't, also great. The goal isn't to produce a geyser—it's to enjoy the journey of pleasure, with or without a splash. So, take the pressure off, lean into what feels good, and let your only measure of success be how much fun you have along the way.

LESSON FORTY-FIVE

WHY SIXTY-NINE IS THE WORLD'S SEXIEST NUMBER (OR IS IT?)

SIXTY-NINE—THE number that launched a thousand memes, inspired a million giggles, and somehow remains one of the most debated sexual positions of all time. For some, it's the pinnacle of mutual pleasure. For others, it's an overhyped balancing act that ends in neck strain and existential regret.

So, how do you make it *actually* enjoyable? Let's break it down.

SIXTY-NINE THROUGH THE AGES: A LONG HISTORY OF ORAL ACROBATICS

Think 69 is a modern invention? Hardly. This entwined pleasure pose has been around for centuries. The Kama Sutra—India's ancient manual of love and sex—features a version of the position, calling it "The Congress of the Crow." The French, ever poetic, coined soixante-neuf (sixty-nine) as a term in the late 18th century, proving their flair for both romance and mathematics.

Erotic art from ancient Greece to Imperial China depicts couples indulging in mutual oral pleasure, highlighting that the struggle to *actually* make this position work is millennia old.

THE COITAL CONUNDRUM

In theory, sixty-nine is the pinnacle of mutual pleasure—two lovers, entwined, simultaneously giving and receiving oral sex. A perfect erotic yin-yang. In reality? Well, it's a logistical puzzle requiring flexibility, coordination, and a certain willingness to embrace the absurd.

For some, the idea of experiencing pleasure while focusing on delivering it is a delightful challenge. For others, it's akin to rubbing your stomach while patting your head—only, you know, with genitals involved. Add height differentials, neck strain, and the pressure to synchronize orgasms, and you might find yourself questioning whether this erotic ouroboros is truly the holy grail of oral sex.

So how do you ensure your experience leans more "hot" than "horrifically uncomfortable?"

PRO TIPS FOR A SMOOTH RIDE

Choose your position wisely. Traditional 69 (stacked, with one partner on top) can be physically demanding—especially for the one on top. Instead, try a side-lying variation. This keeps things intimate, reduces strain, and allows for better control over rhythm and pressure. Bonus: it frees up your hands for extra exploration.

Communication = better orgasms. If something isn't working—angle, speed, depth—say so! A simple moan, hum, or light touch can help guide your partner without breaking the mood. Nonverbal cues are your best friend here.

Slow down and sync up. It's easy to get distracted when giving *and* receiving at the same time. The solution? Pace yourself. Take turns slowing down, letting one partner focus more on pleasure while the other focuses on giving.

Support your body (and your neck). A strategically placed pillow or wedge can work wonders—especially if height difference is an issue. If you're on top, don't hover in a squat (your thighs *will* start burning). Instead, settle in comfortably and adjust your movements so they feel effortless, not like a CrossFit workout.

Focus on more than just the main event. Oral is the star of the show, but don't ignore hands, breath, and touch. Light teasing, playful nibbling, or using your hands to explore can heighten sensation and make everything feel more connected.

IS SIXTY-NINE THE WORLD'S SEXIEST NUMBER?

For some, absolutely. For others, not so much. The truth? *It depends on how you do it.* With a little creativity, some strategic adjustments, and a sense of humor, sixty-nine can be a pleasure-filled, laugh-out-loud, deeply intimate experience. And if it's not for you? No worries—there are plenty of other delicious ways to play.

LESSON FORTY-SIX

MENTAL FOREPLAY: WHY DAYDREAMING IS YOUR SEXIEST SUPERPOWER

LET ME ASK YOU SOMETHING. When was the last time you let your mind wander—*really* wander? Not to your grocery list, not to whether you paid that bill, and definitely not to an imaginary argument with Carol from accounting. I mean the good kind of wandering—the kind that makes you feel *alive*.

If it's been a while, don't worry. Your sexy, radiant, untamed imagination didn't disappear—it just needs a little seduction.

THE LOST ART OF DAYDREAMING (AND WHY YOU NEED IT BACK)

Remember being a kid, staring out the window in math class, lost in a world where you were a rock star, a movie heroine, or the main character in an epic romance? You weren't bored; you were *somewhere else*. Daydreaming was effortless.

Then life happened. The world told you to be productive, to stay focused, to stop "wasting time." And just like that, the wild, juicy, *limitless* part of your imagination took a back seat. But here's the secret: daydreaming isn't frivolous—it's *fuel*. It's the key to reclaiming your sensuality, your creativity, and your desire.

A PERSONAL EXAMPLE (OR, HOW DURAN DURAN CHANGED MY LIFE)

Let me take you back to the 1980s. Picture a mall. A fountain. Me, fresh out of Claire's with blue mascara and a side ponytail. And there, standing just feet away—Simon Le Bon, John Taylor, and (because I'm generous) Nick Rhodes of *Duran Duran*.

In my daydream, I *owned* the scene. I was magnetic. Simon and John both wanted to take me on a date. A dramatic, swoon-worthy tussle ensued.

Now, was this realistic? Not even close. Did it make me feel amazing? *Absolutely.* I can still see myself in the entire daydream—even decades later. And that's the magic: in our daydreams, we are always desired, always confident, always the main character.

HOW TO USE DAYDREAMING TO REKINDLE YOUR INNER SEXY

1. **Rewrite Your Desire Script.** If your fantasies have been on autopilot (or worse, missing entirely), it's time to shake things up. Picture yourself in a setting that excites you—a candlelit hotel room, a moonlit beach, backstage at a concert. Imagine what happens next. Who's there? What's being whispered in your ear? Let the scene unfold *without* self-judgment.
2. **Use It as Mental Foreplay.** Desire starts *before* the bedroom. If you're in a relationship, daydream about your partner *as if they were someone new.* Imagine seeing them across a crowded room, locking eyes like strangers meeting for the first time. That shift in perspective alone can reignite attraction.

3. **Tap Into Your Fantasy Confidence**. Your brain believes what you tell it. Daydream yourself into that *Oh, she's stunning* energy. Walk through your fantasy world *owning* the room, the moment, the pleasure. Confidence isn't just about looks—it's about presence.

4. **Indulge in Sensory Fantasies.** Not all fantasies have to be plot-driven. Imagine the *feeling* of silk sheets on your skin, the slow burn of anticipation, the brush of warm breath against your neck. Engage all your senses—taste, touch, scent, sound, and sight—to make your daydreams deeply immersive.

5. **Make It a Habit**. The more you let yourself daydream, the easier it becomes. Set aside a few minutes a day—maybe in the shower, before bed, or during your afternoon coffee—to let your mind roam. The best part? No one has to know you're doing it.

YOUR INNER SEXY STARTS IN YOUR MIND

Desire, creativity, confidence—it *all* begins upstairs. So stop waiting for permission. Close your eyes, take a deep breath, and slip into the best daydream of your life.

And if anyone knows Simon Le Bon, let's just say… my mind is *very* open.

LESSON FORTY-SEVEN

BLUSH, BEG, BURN: THE THRILL OF HUMILIATION

LET'S talk about a kink that might make you raise an eyebrow and cross your legs—humiliation. That's right, the very thing that haunted your middle school years has become a deliciously complex and wildly arousing playground for some. Stay with me here. Before you recoil at the thought of reliving your seventh-grade embarrassment in the bedroom, let's unravel why this power play is a turn-on, how to navigate it safely, and, most importantly, how to keep the blush on your cheeks from veering into actual emotional distress.

HUMILIATION AS AN EROTIC ART FORM

Humiliation play isn't just about name-calling or verbal degradation; it's a psychological dance, an intricate push-pull of power, vulnerability, and arousal. It's the unexpected thrill of being told what to do, the rush of surrendering control, the whispered reminder that you're not the one in charge tonight. For some, it's an elaborate role-playing game—teacher-student, boss-employee, or any scenario where power dynamics ignite a spark.

And while movies like *Baby Girl* and *Secretary* have brought this kink into mainstream conversation, they're far from its origin. Erotic humiliation has been a part of human desire for centuries, appearing in ancient texts, Victorian-era underground literature, and even the elaborate courtly games of power and submission played by aristocrats. The thrill of being put in one's place—whether through words, posture, or symbolic restraint—is nothing new. It's simply the latest flavor of an old, deeply wired pleasure dynamic.

Unlike full-time dominant/submissive lifestyles, humiliation kinks often exist in isolated play sessions—contained, curated, and, most importantly, completely consensual. It's about stepping into a fantasy for a moment, then stepping back out, dignity still intact.

WHY WE GET OFF ON BEING KNOCKED DOWN (IN THE RIGHT WAY)

Humiliation play stirs up a heady mix of emotions—shame, excitement, submission, and thrill—all rolled into a single, electrifying cocktail. It's no coincidence that those who spend their days commanding boardrooms or fixing crises often fantasize about surrendering in the bedroom. Power reversal can be deeply liberating.

It also plays into the human fascination with the taboo. We spend our lives avoiding shame—never wanting to look foolish in public, never wanting to be called out. But in a safe, structured space, we can flirt with the edges of embarrassment without actual consequences. It's a controlled burn, a way to touch the flame without getting scorched.

THE RULES OF PLAY: HOW TO HUMILIATE WITHOUT HARM

Humiliation play is *not* about tearing someone down—it's about building erotic tension within a trusted, playful framework. Here's how to make it safe, sexy, and satisfying:

- **Consent Is King (or Queen, or Tramp, or Whatever Title Thrills You).** Set clear boundaries before diving in. What's hot? What's off-limits? What words are arousing, and which will ruin the mood? No guessing games—clarity is sexy.
- **Safe Words Save You.** Even if you love the idea of being "punished," you need an emergency escape hatch. A simple "red" means stop, "yellow" means slow down, and "green" means keep going (and maybe go harder). Some people like to get creative—I've heard safe words ranging from "pineapple" to "onomatopoeia" (a bold choice under pressure). Regardless of the word, the dominant partner *must* check in regularly.
- **Aftercare Isn't Optional.** A scene is a scene, and when "cut" is called, you need to transition back to reality. Aftercare—cuddling, chocolate, debriefing, or even just a reassuring word—ensures that everyone leaves the experience feeling good.

HOW TO INTRODUCE HUMILIATION INTO YOUR SEX LIFE

Whether you're brand new to this kink or looking to refine your skills, here are a few ways to make humiliation play work for you.

1. Start Small and Playful. If you're just dipping a toe into the world of humiliation, begin with light teasing. A playful scolding, a denied orgasm, or a well-timed *tsk-tsk* can introduce the dynamic without overwhelming your partner.

2. Use a Mix of Praise and Teasing. Balance is key. Many enjoy being called names (babygirl, brat, slut), but it can be even hotter when combined with praise: "Look at my good girl, begging for it." It's the contrast between shame and validation that makes it intoxicating.

3. Make It Interactive. Have your partner beg for

permission, repeat a phrase, or hold a position while you draw out the anticipation. The more involved they are in their "humiliation," the more arousing the experience.

4. Take It Beyond Words. Verbal degradation isn't the only form of humiliation play. Forced eye contact, being told not to move, wearing something deliberately revealing—humiliation can be sensory and physical as much as verbal.

5. Keep It Playful, Not Personal. The biggest mistake in humiliation play? Crossing the emotional line. Keep criticism sexy, not cutting. "You're such a desperate little thing" works—"I've never met anyone as pathetic as you" does *not*. Know the difference.

FINAL THOUGHTS: KEEP IT HOT, NOT HURTFUL

At the end of the day, humiliation play is about trust, thrill, and pushing just the right buttons. Done well, it's an intoxicating mix of surrender and excitement. Done poorly, and you've got yourself an awkward therapy session waiting to happen.

So go forth, my gorgeous one. Tease. Beg. Blush. Just remember—humiliation should make you weak in the knees, not weak in the heart.

LESSON FORTY-EIGHT

YOUR FIRST SOLO TRIP TO BOOTAY-VILLE— A BEGINNER'S GUIDE TO ANAL MASTURBATION

Are you ready to explore something new and perhaps a little daring? Let's dive into the fascinating world of anal masturbation—a trend that has been rising in popularity (it was named a top sex trend in both 2023 and 2024—yup, that's someone's job). So, yes, it's a thing. And no, you don't need a donut to enjoy it (though the internet seems obsessed with using donuts as metaphors for all things "butt").

But why the fuss? Let's start with the basics: anal masturbation is the self-stimulation of the anus, rectum, and, for those with prostates, the prostate itself, all for the purpose of pleasure. This activity is rich with potential because the anus has a treasure trove of nerve endings that can be incredibly stimulating for people of all genders.

Feeling intrigued? Nervous? Maybe both? That's totally okay. Many of us weren't taught much about regular masturbation, let alone anal self-play. So let's clear the air (pun intended) and dive into some essentials.

WHY EXPLORE ANAL MASTURBATION?

The anus is a hidden gem of pleasure, thanks to its dense network of nerve endings. For people with vulvas, anal stimulation can even indirectly engage the vaginal canal and clitoral structure—neighbors sharing a wall, if you will. But let's be clear: this is a judgment-free zone. If you try it and it's not for you, that's perfectly fine. The goal is to understand your body better, expand your horizons, and discover what brings you joy.

GROUND RULES FOR SAFE EXPLORATION

Before you knock, knock, knock on your backdoor, here's what you need to know:

- **Preparation Is Everything.** Relaxation and arousal are key. Treat this as an occasion—not a quick experiment between Zoom calls. Warm baths and candles can set the mood, while a little external self-play helps your body get ready for the experience.

- **Cleanliness Is Sexy.** Start with clean hands and (I can't stress this enough) trimmed, filed nails. The anus has its own delicate ecosystem, so keeping things clean prevents irritation or infection. Wash your toys thoroughly and avoid anything sharp or porous.

- **Lube Is Your Best Friend.** The anus doesn't self-lubricate, so a good-quality silicone or water-based lubricant is essential. Skip the glittery or scented varieties—your anus really doesn't need extra flair.

- **Start Slow.** Begin with external stimulation before considering penetration. Gentle circles, light pressure, and a mindful pace are key. If you decide

to try insertion, work your way up gradually with
small, anal-safe toys or fingers.

THREE TIPS FOR MAKING ANAL MASTURBATION A THING

- **Get the Right Gear.** Toys labeled as "anal-safe"
  are a must. This means they have a flared base or a
  retrieval loop to prevent any accidental
  disappearances (because no one wants to explain that
  ER visit). If using fingers, make sure nails are short
  and smooth to avoid any unwanted scratches.
- **Experiment with Sensation Before
  Penetration.** Not all anal play has to involve
  insertion. The nerve endings around the anus are
  extremely sensitive, meaning light external
  stimulation—gentle rubbing, circling, or even light
  tapping—can be just as pleasurable. Try teasing
  the area with a vibrator or warming lube to build
  anticipation.
- **Breathe and Let Go.** Tension is the number-one
  mood killer when it comes to anal play. If you're
  holding your breath or clenching, it's going to feel
  more awkward than amazing. Deep, relaxed
  breathing can make a world of difference. Take
  your time, exhale, and let your body ease into the
  sensation.

TROUBLESHOOTING COMMON CHALLENGES

If it's not feeling great, consider these adjustments:

- **Use More Lube**: You can never have enough.
  Truly.

- **Relax and Breathe**: Deep, diaphragmatic breaths can ease tension and make the experience more enjoyable.
- **Adjust Positioning**: Experiment with positions like lying on your back with a pillow under your hips or on all fours to find what feels best.

THE BOTTOM LINE

Anal masturbation isn't for everyone, and that's perfectly okay. If you're curious, approach it with patience, humor, and an open mind. Think of this as an adventure—not a check list item to win any sexploration contests. Whether it's a one-time experiment or a new favorite, you're taking another step toward understanding and embracing your body's potential for pleasure. Happy exploring!

LESSON FORTY-NINE

COSPLAY SEX—THE BENEFITS OF GETTING IT ON IN CHARACTER

Are you ready to step into a new role . . . and out of your everyday skin? Imagine slipping into a character—not just a costume—and discovering a playful, untapped version of yourself. Welcome to the world of cosplay, where creativity meets connection, and yes, the bedroom becomes a stage for passion (I said that in a fantastic accent!).

Cosplay, short for "costume play," originated in 1984 when Nobuyuki Takahashi first coined the term in a Japanese magazine. While its roots lie in sci-fi conventions, today, cosplay has expanded into a form of self-expression—and a surprisingly sexy way to shake things up.

WHY COSPLAY WORKS: LESSONS FROM PLAY AND PERFORMANCE

Children instinctively understand the magic of dress-up. It's transformative, freeing, and a confidence booster. Adults can channel this same energy. When you put on a costume, you're not just adorning your body—you're stepping into a different mindset. Theater performers and drag queens know this intimately; the costume is an invitation to embody a character fully.

And here's the sexy part: by exploring new roles, you can unlock boldness and fantasies that may feel out of reach in your everyday persona. Cosplay isn't about perfection—it's about permission.

THE SEXY SIDE OF COSPLAY

Cosplay creates a space for curiosity and experimentation. Whether you're in a long-term relationship, newly exploring love, or even flying solo, this practice opens doors to:

- **Confidence.** Embodying a character can help you feel powerful and seductive. And newness is a dopamine booster, which is the pleasure neurotransmitter!
- **Connection.** Sharing fantasies through play deepens intimacy.
- **Creativity.** The process of choosing and becoming a character is as thrilling as the act itself.

Imagine yourself as Wonder Woman with her lasso of truth or a rogue pirate captain on the high seas. It's not just role-play; it's a dynamic way to shed inhibitions and explore your desires. And the possibilities are endless.

THREE TIPS FOR TAKING COSPLAY FROM CUTE TO CLIMAX

- **Get Inspired and Plan Ahead.** Half the fun of cosplay is the buildup. Find inspiration from movies, books, or even video games. Pinterest boards, online forums, and Reddit threads dedicated to cosplay are treasure troves of ideas. Don't just think about the costume—think about the scenario. Are you a captured spy? A Jedi with *needs*? A librarian about to deliver *punishments* for overdue books? The more detail, the hotter the experience.

- **Keep It Low-Stress and High-Reward.** Cosplay sex isn't about a Hollywood-level costume budget. If you want to go all out, great! But a small detail—a mask, a prop, a pair of thigh-high boots—can transform the mood just as effectively. If the idea of a full costume feels overwhelming, ease in with partial role-play, like taking on a seductive new persona (British accent optional, but encouraged).

- **Play the Part—Not Just Wear It.** A corset alone doesn't make you a temptress. A cape doesn't make you a villain. *Embody* the character. How would they talk? Move? Tease? This is where cosplay shifts from "fun dress-up" to full-body immersion. Don't be afraid to throw in a little storytelling—narratives can be powerful aphrodisiacs.

TRY CLASSIC POWER-DYNAMIC DUOS

If you don't know where to start, opt for tried-and-true pairings that naturally create tension:

- **Pirate and captive**—because who doesn't love a little swashbuckling foreplay?
- **Detective and suspect**—where interrogations get *intimate.*
- **Royalty and servant**—for a night of decadent indulgence.
- **Sci-fi adventurers**—think Han and Leia, but with *less* bickering (or more, if that's your thing).
- **Superhero and villain**—because someone *always* gets tied up.

DON'T SKIP THE AFTERCARE

Cosplay can be an intense experience, especially if it involves power play. After the fun, take a moment to check in, transition back to reality, and maybe laugh about how ridiculous yet amazing it was. Snuggle, debrief, or—if you went full method actor—celebrate your *Best Performance in a Leading Role* with a well-earned drink.

WHERE TO FIND COSTUMES THAT WON'T BREAK THE BANK

You don't need a Comic-Con budget to bring a character to life. Thrift stores, Halloween pop-ups, and online shops like Etsy and Dolls Kill have affordable, sexy options. Even repurposing something from your closet—say, an oversized buttondown as a "borrowed" piece from your *very* naughty professor —can work wonders. And don't forget accessories! A simple mask or a pair of gloves can be just as transformative as a full-blown costume.

THE EMOTIONAL PAYOFF

Cosplay isn't just about sex—it's about rediscovering joy and imagination. It reduces anxiety, boosts dopamine, and reminds us that play is a form of intimacy. By stepping into a character, you're not escaping reality; you're enhancing it.

So, grab that cape, crown, or lasso (or all three). The bedroom is your stage, and the script is yours to write. Step into your role and live sexily ever after—in character.

LESSON FIFTY

CUCKOO FOR CUCKOLDING? WHY THIS KINK IS MAKING A SURPRISING COMEBACK

Ah, cuckolding—a word that lands with the weight of medieval tragedy yet whispers of modern erotic intrigue. If you feel a little "cucky" today, rest assured, you are in historic company. This practice, with its roots entangled in literature, myth, and gender politics, has been resurrected from the annals of shame into an arena of consensual desire. And yes, it is making quite the comeback.

FROM CHAUCER TO CLICKBAIT: A BRIEF HISTORY

Cuckolding is old—very old. The term itself derives from the cuckoo bird, notorious for laying its eggs in another bird's nest, outsourcing the burden of parenthood. In medieval literature, the cuckold was the unwitting fool, his wife's infidelity a cause for village-wide amusement. Shakespeare milked it for dramatic despair, while the Trojan War itself—let's be honest—was basically a military campaign over a cuckolded king's bruised ego.

By the eighteenth century, the term had all but vanished. Perhaps the stiff moral codes of Victorian prudery rendered the discussion of spousal straying a bit too, well, impolite. But like flared jeans and vinyl records, what is old is new again.

And cuckolding, once the insult *du jour*, has found fresh life in the realm of erotic exploration.

THE MODERN CUCKOLD: NOT SO UNWITTING AFTER ALL

Fast forward to today, and cuckolding is no longer just the stuff of whispered gossip and scandalous affairs. Now, it is a consensual practice, often within otherwise monogamous relationships. Unlike its historic counterpart, the modern cuckold is not an oblivious fool but an active participant—one who delights in the arousal of his (or her) partner's escapades.

For many, cuckolding flips the script on possession and power, transforming old narratives of humiliation into ones of erotic liberation. It sits at the intersection of dominance and submission, of control and surrender, of taboo and titillation. And, intriguingly, studies suggest that this particular fantasy is disproportionately appealing to conservative men. The irony is just . . . delicious.

WHY IS CUCKOLDING SO AROUSING?

At its core, cuckolding is about transgression. It is about stepping outside the script of monogamy and reveling in the very thing society warns against. The jealousy, the thrill of the forbidden, the vulnerability—it all heightens arousal.

There is also an element of eroticized contrast. The cuckold, by design, is confronted with the image of their partner with another—often someone younger, stronger, more virile (in cuckold lore, called "the bull"). And yet, rather than eroding intimacy, many couples claim it fosters deeper communication, trust, and connection. Like all kinks, it thrives on boundaries and consent.

THREE TIPS FOR LIVING SEXILY EVER AFTER WITH CUCKOLD ENERGY

Whether you are into this kink or just intrigued by the themes of power, surrender, and voyeurism, here's how to take its best elements and apply them to your own erotic life:

1. **Use the Power of Erotic Storytelling.** Even if actual cuckolding is not your thing, the idea of narrating a fantasy or indulging in role-play can ignite new levels of intimacy. Describe a scenario to your partner, send a provocative voice memo, or exchange steamy texts that push your boundaries in a safe way.

2. **Redefine What "Cheating" Means for You.** Monogamy is not *one-size-fits-all.* Many couples explore ethical non-monogamy, voyeurism, or simply a more open dialogue about attraction without crossing any physical lines. The key is trust —when both partners feel secure, curiosity can become an asset instead of a threat.

3. **Play with Power and Permission.** One reason cuckolding is so alluring is that it shifts the traditional power dynamic. Even if you are not into the full kink, you can explore elements of control and surrender through BDSM, role-play, or even something as simple as a partner "granting permission" to flirt in social settings.

THE FINAL ACT: PLAY, DON'T PANIC

Cuckolding may not be for everyone, but it invites a larger conversation about sexual freedom, trust, and the narratives we inherit about fidelity and ownership. Maybe for you, the idea is an instant turn-off. Maybe it's a thrilling fantasy. Or maybe, just maybe, it's one of those things best left to the imagination—where it can be just as powerful, just as provocative, and just as deliciously taboo.

Whatever your take, remember: the key to a fulfilling erotic life isn't following the rules. It's about writing your own. Oh, wow . . . that almost sounded downright Shakespearean!

LESSON FIFTY-ONE

TO VAB OR NOT TO VAB? THE SEXY SCIENCE OF SEDUCTION

WE'RE ABOUT to dive into one of the spiciest, most eyebrow-raising seduction methods to hit the mainstream: vabbing.

Now, I usually take viral trends with a grain of salt (and maybe a sip of something spicy), but when a dear patient over 40 asked me, "Should I be doing this?" well, darling, we had to go there.

VABBING: WHAT IS IT? AND SHOULD YOU TRY IT?

Vabbing—a blend of "vaginal" and "dabbing"—is the art of applying your own vaginal fluids to pulse points like the wrists and behind the ears in hopes of attracting a mate. It's marketed as your own personal pheromone perfume, a scent that supposedly triggers primal attraction.

But before you start bottling your essence, let's get scientific. Pheromones are chemical signals that influence behavior among the same species. In animals, they play a crucial role in mating. But here's the twist: after decades of research, scientists have yet to confirm that humans even produce pheromones in the same way.

So, is vabbing a seductive superpower or just wishful thinking? Science isn't sold on the idea, but psychology might be. Because here's the real magic: confidence is intoxicating. The sheer act of vabbing—your secret weapon—might just put you in a mindset of boldness, flirtation, and self-assurance. And that, my love, is sex appeal in its purest form.

THE DO'S AND DON'TS OF VABBING

If you're vabbing-curious (and I know you are), let's establish some golden rules:

- **Hygiene is everything.** Wash your hands before and after. Your delicate ecosystem deserves nothing less.
- **Consent, always.** Your vabbed wrists should not be rubbing up against unsuspecting gym-goers. Let's keep it classy, please.
- **Listen to your body.** If something smells "off," it's time to check in with your gyno, not your dating app.

THREE TIPS FOR VABBING LIKE A PRO

1. **Pair It with a Ritual.** Confidence isn't about a scent; it's about how you carry yourself. Set an intention before you vab—whether it's to exude allure, spark a flirty conversation, or just feel like an absolute goddess. Combine it with a spritz of your favorite perfume, a power stance, or that dress that makes you feel invincible.
2. **Use It as a Mindset Shift.** The power of vabbing isn't necessarily in the smell—it's in the act. When you engage in a private ritual, you move through the world differently. Walk into a room with the energy that you're a rare, intoxicating experience (because, spoiler alert: you are).

3. **Keep It Playful.** Vabbing is not a magic spell, but it *is* an invitation to explore your own erotic energy. Try it on a first date, at a party, or even just to test your own reaction. Treat it as an experiment, not an obligation. If it makes you feel amazing, fabulous. If not, no harm done— confidence is the real seduction technique, and you already have that in spades.

THE BOTTOM LINE

So, should you vab? If it makes you feel more embodied, more playful, and more *you*—why not? The real allure isn't in the scent itself but in the intention behind it. And that, my love, is the secret to living sexily ever after.

Vab away, or don't. Either way, you're already irresistible.

LESSON FIFTY-TWO

EROTIC HYPNOSIS—THE SEXY MIND HACK YOU DIDN'T KNOW YOU NEEDED

Hypnosis—it's not just for quitting smoking or clucking like a chicken at a bachelorette party. Erotic hypnosis is an entirely different beast, one where pleasure starts in the mind before it even reaches the body. Welcome to the world of erotic hypnosis, where ancient science meets modern seduction. And spoiler alert: your brain is your biggest erogenous zone.

WHAT EROTIC HYPNOSIS IS (AND ISN'T)

Before you picture some stage magician snapping his fingers and commanding you to undress, let's set the record straight: erotic hypnosis isn't about mind control or anything nonconsensual. It's a guided journey into deep relaxation, where your conscious mind takes a backseat and your sensual self emerges. Whether you want to enhance pleasure, overcome sexual hurdles, or just explore something new, this is about tuning into your own desire—not someone else's commands.

And yes, if you're curious, there are some wildly talented hypnotherapists demonstrating their skills (with consenting participants) on YouTube.

WHY TRY EROTIC HYPNOSIS?

1. **Unlock Deeper Pleasure**: Ever feel like you *should* be enjoying sex more, but something's holding you back? Erotic hypnosis helps rewire the brain for pleasure, letting you drop those mental blocks and experience sex fully—without distractions.

2. **Boost Libido (Without a Pill)**: Life is exhausting. Stress, hormones, and sheer overwhelm can kill desire faster than bad lighting. Hypnosis reconnects your mind and body so that getting in the mood isn't just something you *schedule*—it's something you *want*.

3. **Explore Fantasies—Safely**: Ever had a fantasy that intrigued you but wasn't something you wanted to act on in real life? Hypnosis lets you play it out vividly, all in your head—no logistics, no contracts, no awkward cleanup.

4. **Turn Up the Orgasm Dial**: Your brain controls how you experience pleasure. Erotic hypnosis can heighten sensations, extend orgasms, or even induce hands-free climaxes (yes, that's a thing). Some women report multiple orgasms for the first time after hypnosis.

5. **Confidence, Darling. Confidence:** If self-doubt has ever whispered *You're not sexy enough* in your ear, hypnosis is your comeback. It helps rewrite those old scripts, replacing insecurity with full-body goddess energy.

6. **Kink Without Commitment**: Curious about BDSM but not ready to dive in? Hypnosis can mimic the mental effects of submission, dominance, and surrender—without a single rope or blindfold in sight.

7. **The Ultimate Mental Foreplay**: Think of erotic hypnosis as preheating the oven. It builds arousal, anticipation, and surrender *before* anything physical even starts—meaning by the time you do get to the main event, your mind is already primed for pleasure.

HOW TO TRY IT

Not all hypnotherapists specialize in erotic hypnosis, so look for sex-positive professionals trained in both hypnotherapy and sexual wellness. A few great places to start:

- **The American Association of Sexuality Educators, Counselors, and Therapists (AASECT)** – www.aasect.org
- **The Society for Clinical and Experimental Hypnosis (SCEH)** – www.sceh.us

If you're intrigued by the idea of deepening intimacy, heightening pleasure, or exploring fantasies in a whole new way, erotic hypnosis might just be your next favorite adventure. Consider it a tune-up for your erotic mind—because pleasure starts *between your ears* long before it reaches anywhere else.

LESSON FIFTY-THREE

PEGGING—HOW THIS PLUG-AND-PLAY KINK IS ROYALLY AMAZING

LET'S TALK ABOUT PEGGING—A bold, boundary-expanding adventure in intimacy. For the uninitiated, pegging involves anal penetration using a strap-on, often flipping traditional roles of giver and receiver. But this isn't just about physical sensation; it's an invitation to explore trust, vulnerability, and connection on a deeper level. And let's be real—everyone looks hot in a strap-on.

WHY PEGGING MATTERS

Pegging is more than just a kinky detour—it's a playful reimagining of power dynamics, pleasure, and connection. It challenges the idea that one person always gives and the other always receives, making room for fluidity, curiosity, and, let's face it, some mind-blowing sensations. For the giver, it's an empowering, playful shift in control. For the receiver, it's an opportunity to surrender and experience pleasure in a way that's often overlooked.

And if you think this is a trend confined to the *Fifty Shades* era, think again. Cultures have celebrated anal play for centuries—it's just that modern sex education skipped that chapter. So, let's catch up.

THE ESSENTIALS: PEGGING LIKE A PRO

1. **Lube, Lube, Lube (And Then More Lube)**.
   The anus doesn't self-lubricate, so a silicone or
   water-based lubricant is non-negotiable. Go for the
   good stuff—thicker formulas designed for anal play
   are your best bet. And let's be clear: no one has
   ever regretted using *too much* lube.

2. **Start Small, Build Big**: If you or your partner
   are new to anal play, don't go straight for the
   Excalibur of strap-ons. Start with fingers, external
   stimulation, or beginner-friendly toys to get
   familiar with the sensations. Think of it as
   stretching before a workout—except way more fun.

3. **Strap in, but Make It Comfortable**: A well-
   fitting harness makes all the difference. Look for
   adjustable straps, breathable materials, and a style
   that suits your aesthetic (yes, there are lace-
   trimmed options for when you want to feel dainty
   and deadly). Try it on beforehand and practice
   moving with it—because nothing kills the mood
   like fumbling with buckles mid-action.

4. **Name Your Strap-On**: A little humor goes a
   long way. Naming your strap-on makes the
   experience feel less intimidating and way more fun.
   "Captain Thrust" or "Lady Mjolnir" might be too
   much, but "Trudy" or "Mildred" could bring the
   right amount of cheeky charm to the moment.

5. **Communicate Like You're Landing a Plane**:
   This is a team effort, and like any great adventure,
   clear signals are crucial. Check in before, during,

and after—not in a mood-killing way, but enough to keep both partners feeling good. Also, a reminder for all givers: slow, steady, and *for the love of all things King Arthur,* don't just ram it in.

THE JOY OF ROLE REVERSAL

Pegging flips the script, letting partners step into new roles and explore pleasure from a different angle—literally. For those with prostates, it can unlock a new realm of orgasmic potential. For those who've always been on the receiving end, taking control can be exhilarating.

More importantly, pegging gives permission to *play.* Sex can be serious, but it can also be hilarious, exploratory, and completely unexpected. Whether it becomes a regular thing or a one-time adventure, pegging is about giving yourself the freedom to experience pleasure in ways you never thought possible.

So, grab some lube, find the perfect harness, and remember: in the kingdom of pleasure, everyone deserves the chance to wear the crown.

LESSON FIFTY-FOUR

THE ART OF THE REAR VIEW—ELEVATING DOGGY STYLE BEYOND THE BASICS

Ah, *doggy style*—a position that sounds like it belongs more at a pet adoption event than in a boudoir. Whoever named it was clearly not in charge of marketing. But don't let the branding fool you; this pose is a powerhouse of pleasure, control, and versatility. Whether you're after deep connection, delicious abandon, or just an incredibly flattering angle (yes, it's the waist-snatcher of the bedroom), it's time to elevate this classic from primal grunt to erotic masterpiece.

WHY DOGGY STYLE DESERVES A REBRAND

At its core, this position is about access—G-spot, prostate, or a mix of both, depending on your anatomy. It also allows for a tantalizing power dynamic: the giver controls the thrust, the receiver controls the depth (because trust me, a well-timed push-back is a *statement*). But contrary to its reputation, this position doesn't have to feel detached. It can be intensely intimate, deeply connected, and—depending on the mood—slow, sensual, or just gloriously filthy.

And let's not forget: this position has had some truly *cinematic* moments. Angelina Jolie in *Original Sin*, Cate Blanchett in

Carol, and a million slow-burn love scenes that prove doggy isn't just about speed—it's about style.

FIVE WAYS TO ELEVATE THE REAR-VIEW RENDEZVOUS

1. **Comfort Is Queen.** Let's start with the basics. If you're on your hands and knees, give those joints a break—sex pillows, stacked cushions, or even a rolled-up towel under the knees will keep you from feeling like a medieval peasant after five minutes. Try positioning yourself on all fours but resting your upper body on a soft surface (bed, couch, willing partner's chest). The more supported you are, the longer you'll want to stay in the moment.

2. **Play with Angles for Maximum Pleasure.** Newsflash: not all doggy styles are created equal. A subtle shift in position can completely change the experience. If you tilt your hips upward (think Instagram-worthy arch), it increases G-spot stimulation. Flattening your torso against the bed? That deepens penetration and creates a grinding effect. Want to keep things closer? Have the giver bring their knees together to limit movement for a tighter, more controlled experience.

3. **Hands, Mouth, and Everything Else.** Just because you're facing away doesn't mean connection is off the table. Reach back and guide their hands to your waist, thighs, or anywhere else you want attention. If you're in front, use your own hands for clitoral stimulation or add a toy into the mix. Bonus: mirrors. Because seeing yourself in action is its *own* kind of turn-on.

4. **Rhythm Rules the Game.** Doggy style isn't just about thrusting at the speed of a poorly tuned

jackhammer. A well-timed pause, a shift in rhythm, or a deep, slow grind can turn this from good to mind-blowing. Change it up—fast, slow, teasing, holding still while someone else moves. The best music builds to a crescendo, not a sudden crash landing.

5. **Bring in the Extras.** Want to really mix things up? Try incorporating a blindfold, a well-placed smack, or even a bit of hair-pulling (gently, we all like to keep what's left). Add a vibrating plug for extra stimulation or a whispered command that makes you blush. Doggy doesn't have to be all grunts and sweat—it can be a slow, seductive tease, too.

REDEFINING DOGGY STYLE: MAKE IT YOUR OWN

Forget what you've been told—doggy style isn't just for one type of lover, one speed, or one experience. It can be elegant, intimate, and deeply satisfying when done with intention. So tilt a little higher, adjust a little lower, and remember: every rear-view deserves a little *art direction*.

And when in doubt, remember this: every doggy has its day.

LESSON FIFTY-FIVE

THE YONI MASSAGE—A MASTERCLASS IN RECEIVING

Ah, Tantra. I like to say it the way I imagine Sting does—*Taaahhn-trahhh*. The ancient practice of slowing down, breathing deeply, and treating pleasure not as a fleeting act but as a *state of being*. And nestled within this wisdom is something deeply sacred, sensual, and—let's be honest—overdue for mainstream appreciation: the yoni massage.

Let's clear something up immediately: a yoni massage is *not* a frantic race to the finish line. It is not a "quick-release" kind of situation. The Sanskrit word *yoni* translates to sacred space, and that's exactly how it should be treated. This isn't about performance or proving anything—it's about reconnecting with yourself, unraveling tension, and learning to *receive*. And, if you choose, deepening intimacy with a partner in a way that feels both ancient and entirely new.

THE YONI KNOWS THINGS

Much like its counterpart, the lingam massage (a practice for those with penises), the yoni massage is an intentional journey that moves through full-body relaxation, breathwork, and deeply attuned touch—from the thighs, to the belly, to the breasts, to *everywhere* in between.

But this is more than just a feel-good indulgence. The yoni holds stories. It holds tension, stress, repression—sometimes even unspoken grief. If you've ever clenched your jaw at a frustrating email, you can bet your yoni has done the same. A yoni massage is about release—not just physically, but emotionally. It's a way to unravel old patterns, invite pleasure without pressure, and rewire the way you experience intimacy.

WHY EVERY WOMAN SHOULD EXPERIENCE A YONI MASSAGE AT LEAST ONCE

Yes, it feels incredible. But beyond the pleasure, here's what it offers:

- **Emotional Release** – You might cry. You might laugh. You might feel an unexpected wave of peace. The body remembers things the mind has long forgotten, and this practice allows them to surface and soften.
- **A Sensual Reset** – Whether you're flying solo or exploring with a partner, a yoni massage can help you understand what *actually* feels good—on your own terms, without external expectations.
- **Mind-Body Reconnection** – We spend so much time living from the neck up, caught in to-do lists and responsibilities. This practice brings you back into your body, moment by moment.
- **Enhanced Intimacy** – For couples, giving (or receiving) a yoni massage isn't just about sex—it's about trust, patience, and deepening physical and emotional connection.

HOW TO MAKE IT AN EXPERIENCE WORTH REPEATING

- **Set the Scene Like the Queen You Are.** This isn't a *Netflix and absentminded touching* kind of moment. This is an event. Set the mood with soft blankets, flickering candles, and a playlist of something sultry but wordless (because nothing kills a mood like a rogue Ed Sheeran lyric). Essential oils like jasmine, lavender, or sandalwood can be luxurious—just don't *actually* put them *in* the yoni. This is about ambiance, not an impromptu science experiment.
- **Slow Everything Way, Way Down.** If you think you're going slow, go even slower. This is about savoring every sensation, not rushing to the "main event." Start with breathwork—deep belly breaths that signal to your nervous system that it's time to relax. If you're with a partner, synchronize breathing to deepen the connection.
- **Focus on the Entire Body, Not Just the Obvious Spots**. The thighs, lower belly, hips, and inner arms are rich with sensitivity. Explore without agenda—this isn't a direct road to orgasm (though if that happens, fabulous). It's about exploration, teasing out tension, and simply *feeling*. If you're with a partner, let them know what feels good *without pressure*. And if you're solo? Luxuriate in your own touch.
- **Release the Pressure to Perform**. Women are often the givers—of love, time, energy. But when was the last time you allowed yourself to *receive*? A yoni massage is about reclaiming pleasure without the obligation to reciprocate. It's not about how

you *look*; it's about how you *feel*. This is a *zero-pressure zone*.

- **Let the Body Lead.** Whether solo or partnered, trust the signals of your own body. Maybe it wants light feathering touch; maybe it wants deep, grounding pressure. Maybe it just wants a moment to rest. There's no *right* way to do this—there's only *your* way.

THE ART OF RECEIVING—YOUR PLEASURE, YOUR BIRTHRIGHT

Pleasure is not a luxury. It's not something you *earn* after a long day of ticking boxes off a list. It is your birthright. The yoni massage is an invitation—to reclaim, to relax, to rediscover. Whether with a trusted partner, a professional, or your own hands, let this be the moment where you learn to *fully receive*.

So tonight, light the freakin' candles. Take a deep breath. And remind yourself: your pleasure is not an afterthought—it's the whole damn story.

LESSON FIFTY-SIX

RIMMING: WHY A LITTLE SALAD TOSSING MIGHT BE YOUR NEW FAVORITE MAIN COURSE

Darling, let's talk about the one meal that doesn't require utensils but does demand a little savoir-faire. Yes, I'm talking about rimming—analingus, the tantalizing tongue-tango that has long been whispered about but rarely given its rightful place at the sexual table.

Maybe you're intrigued, maybe you're horrified, or maybe you're simply salad-curious. Wherever you stand, I invite you to pull up a chair because there's much to discuss. (Cue the French café accordion music.)

WHY IS RIMMING STILL SO TABOO?

We live in an age where we glorify butts—lifting them, sculpting them, even insuring them—but pleasuring them? Mon dieu! The cultural contradictions are delicious. While certain corners of pop culture have been singing its praises (yes, Nicki Minaj, I hear you), many still see rimming as the forbidden fruit of intimacy.

But let's set the record straight: the anus is a nerve-dense pleasure zone, capable of sensations as electrifying as those found elsewhere on the body—if not more. So why does it remain the last frontier? Hygiene fears? A vestigial shame from a puritanical past? The simple truth is that cultural norms often lag behind what our bodies already know: pleasure is pleasure. And when approached with care, curiosity, and good manners (yes, darling, manners always matter), rimming can be a profoundly erotic experience.

THE ETIQUETTE OF ANALINGUS: WHAT EVERY CONNOISSEUR SHOULD KNOW

Before diving tongue-first into this adventure, let's talk about preparation. A fine dining experience requires a pristine table setting, and rimming is no exception.

- **Freshness Is Key.** No one wants old rusty lettuce! A warm shower, a thorough cleanse with gentle soap, and perhaps a shared bathing ritual can turn hygiene into foreplay.
- **Communication, Always.** If this is new territory, express curiosity rather than assumption. "Would you enjoy this?" lands far better than a surprise expedition.
- **Safety Is Sexy.** If you're with a new partner, use a barrier like a dental dam. And always, always remember the golden rule: what visits the back door does not return to the front door.

HOW TO RIM LIKE A SEDUCTIVE GOURMAND

This is not a hurried bite into an apple. This is a slow, sensory experience. Think about licking a glorious ice cream cone— one that thrives on variation.

- Use **light flicks, broad strokes, warm breath, gentle suction**—the full orchestra, not just one lonely kazoo.

- **Tease. Pause. Resume.** The secret to great oral pleasure is anticipation, not mechanics. No one wants just a bunch of hot breath in their booty.
- **Engage the whole body.** Hands, lips, even a well-timed whisper can elevate the experience.

And remember: this is a menu, not a mandate. You don't have to love every dish, but why not taste before deciding?

THREE TIPS TO ELEVATE YOUR RIMMING GAME

1. **Turn the Prep into Foreplay.** A shared shower, a sexy back massage, or a playful "clean-up" session can make the build-up just as fun as the act itself.
2. **Add a Sensory Layer.** Try flavored lubes, warm breath, or a bit of light spanking to heighten the experience.
3. **Switch Up Positions.** The classic bent-over stance isn't your only option. Try lying flat with a pillow under the hips for ultimate relaxation, or sit on the edge of a bed for easier access.

THE BOTTOM LINE (YEP, WENT THERE.)

Pleasure is an expansive landscape, not a rigid map. Some will embrace this exploration eagerly; others may decide it's not for them. Both choices are equally valid. What matters is the willingness to be curious, to explore with intention, and to keep the erotic conversation open.

So, tell me—will you be dining differently tonight?

LESSON FIFTY-SEVEN

POSITION POTPOURRI—THE WEIRD, WACKY, AND WOW-WORTHY MOVES TO TRY AT LEAST ONCE

Hey, you. I see you. You're adventurous, curious, and maybe just a little stuck in your favorite go-to positions. We've all been there—sex ruts happen. And while a classic will always be a classic (hello, missionary and doggy style), sometimes, you need to shake things up, bend a little, stretch a bit, and maybe even defy gravity. Welcome to today's lesson: a sexy buffet of moves that range from sensual to Cirque du Soleil-level acrobatics.

Now, let's get one thing straight—some of these positions are best attempted with a warm-up (think yoga, not just foreplay), and a few may require more enthusiasm than actual execution. But whether you try them in earnest or just giggle about them over cocktails, the goal remains the same: keeping pleasure playful.

WHY SHAKE UP YOUR ROUTINE?

Our bodies are constantly evolving—yes, evolving, not just aging. What worked in our twenties may not be ideal in our fifties, but that doesn't mean we retire our sexual curiosity. If anything, now is the time to explore with confidence, humor, and a little bit of audacity.

Trying new positions can:

- Engage different muscle groups (hello, accidental fitness routine!)
- Intensify intimacy through eye contact and touch
- Offer new angles of stimulation, making old favorites feel brand new

A FEW POSITIONS TO TEMPT YOU

- **The Upstanding Citizen**. Perfect for those who love a little Hollywood drama, this position has one partner standing while the other wraps their legs around them koala-style. Think passionate, wall-slamming, "I must have you now" energy. Pro tip: A sturdy surface for support (hello, kitchen counter or a well-anchored bookshelf) can help keep the moment sexy, not slapstick. Or slapdick, in some cases. Ouch.
- **X Marks the Spot**. If slow and sensual is your speed, this one's for you. Seated facing each other on the bed, you cross your legs over one another, forming an X, and lean back. This isn't about frantic thrusting—it's about deep, lazy grinding, eye contact, and teasing touches. Think of it as the Sunday morning brunch of sex positions—leisurely, indulgent, and best savored slowly.
- **The Pretzel Dip.** A side-lying twist on missionary, one partner lies in a relaxed, classic "Playboy pose" while the other enters from a kneeling position. The result? Deep penetration, comfortable leverage, and a front-row seat to all the delicious facial expressions happening up close and personal.

- **The Spider.** A tangled web of limbs, this one is both visually stunning and functionally fantastic. One partner sits back while the other straddles, leaning in so legs intertwine. It's all about control —grinding, touching, and maximizing clitoral stimulation. Bonus: If you ever wanted to say, "Let's Spider tonight," now's your chance.
- **The Tabletop.** Not to be confused with where you serve dinner—though if you're feeling bold, no judgment! Here, the receiving partner sits on a sturdy surface while the other stands, making this perfect for partners with height differences or those who want a hot, impromptu quickie.
- **The Erotic Accordion.** Reserved for the truly adventurous (and somewhat flexible). The receiving partner squats onto their partner while their partner's legs rest on their shoulders. Yes, it looks as kinky as it sounds, but it offers a uniquely controlled, intimate experience. Plus, it's a great core workout.

THREE TIPS TO AMP UP YOUR POSITION GAME

1. **Turn the Attempt into Foreplay.** Just discussing new positions can spark excitement and anticipation. Browse through an illustrated guide together (or a few steamy romance novels) and pick one to attempt.
2. **Use Props Like a Pro.** A well-placed pillow, a sturdy piece of furniture, or even a sex wedge can make wild positions infinitely more comfortable and accessible. Sometimes, the right angle is just a cushion away.
3. **Laugh, Adjust, Repeat.** If something isn't working, don't force it. Adjust, switch to something

else, or just laugh and roll with it. Some positions sound better in theory than in execution, and that's part of the fun.

FINAL THOUGHT: IT'S ABOUT FUN, NOT PERFECTION

Sex positions are not Olympic events—you don't need perfect form or flawless execution, although a strong dismount (and sticking the landing) is essential. If something doesn't quite work, laugh it off and try another. The key is exploration, playfulness, and finding what brings you pleasure. So go forth, bend a little, twist a lot, and most importantly—enjoy the ride.

LESSON FIFTY-EIGHT

THE BUFFET OF PLEASURE—BEYOND THE BIG THREE

Darling, if you thought sex was limited to the "big three"—vaginal, oral, and anal—then buckle up, because we're about to take a delightful detour through the winding roads of alternative intimacy.

Perhaps you've heard whispers that "everyone is doing it"—whatever "it" is—but let me assure you, sexuality has always been a rich tapestry of exploration. History books and bedrooms alike are filled with unconventional delights, and there's something liberating about knowing that pleasure isn't bound by anatomy, tradition, or expectation.

So why venture beyond the usual? For some, it's the thrill of variety. Others find these acts deepen intimacy, offer practical alternatives to penetrative sex, or work around physical limitations. Whatever the reason, the only rules are consent, comfort, and curiosity.

A TOUR OF THE LESS-TRAVELED EROTIC LANDSCAPES

- **Intermammary Intercourse (a.k.a. Titty F*cking).** Ah, the ever-puzzling, yet ever-popular act of sliding between the breasts. Clinically known as intermammary intercourse, it's been celebrated in erotic literature for centuries. Some women even find it pleasurable if combined with nipple stimulation (hello, nerve pathways to the clitoris!). Is it for everyone? No. But if it piques your curiosity, experiment with angles, positions, and added sensations. Bonus points for a creative name —"Mount Motorboob" has a certain ring to it.

- **Axilism (a.k.a. Armpit Sex).** If you thought armpits were just for deodorant, think again. Some lovers adore the warmth, pressure, and natural musk of axillary intimacy. For some, it's deeply sensual. For others, a mystery best left unsolved. Either way, it's proof that erogenous zones are as much about mindset as mechanics.

- **Outercourse & Dry Humping.** Long before the base system dictated what "counts," dry humping was the MVP of young love. But newsflash: it's not just for teenagers. Grinding against each other, clothed or unclothed, can be thrilling at any age. And as Dr. Ruth always said, outercourse is a valid and safe way to achieve orgasm—no penetration necessary.

- **Buttock Sex & "Sweet Meat" Play.** Think of this as the "in-between pleasure." Using the buttocks or the upper thigh/buttock area (aka the "sweet meat") to create friction is yet another way to enjoy full-body intimacy. It's also a great option for those who want non-penetrative play but still crave skin-on-skin contact.

- **Scissoring & Grinding.** A staple of same-sex intimacy, scissoring is not just a pornographic fantasy—it's real, it's exhilarating, and when done with rhythm and lube, it can be a clitoral symphony. Sure, it takes core strength, coordination, and patience, but when you find your groove, the payoff is spectacular.

- **Fingering & Fisting**. From the delicate tease of a single finger to the deep, exploratory journey of fisting, digital play is versatile and deeply personal. Fingers can navigate angles and pressure points that other tools of pleasure cannot. But remember: lube, patience, and communication are key. And if anyone starts jackhammering away like they're drilling for oil, you need to redirect, educate, and protect the sacred temple that is your body.

THE LESSER-KNOWN ACTS

- **Coitus Interfemoris (between the thighs):** A time-honored technique with minimal risk but maximum friction.
- **Genuflation (knee play):** Who knew knees could be erotic?
- **Foot Jobs:** For lovers of feet and the sensory possibilities they bring.

YOUR PERMISSION SLIP TO EXPLORE

If there's one takeaway, it's this: pleasure is a playground, not a syllabus. You don't have to try everything, but isn't it nice to know you could?

1. **Surprise your partner with something new.** Novelty fuels passion, and a playful spirit keeps the embers glowing.
2. **Communicate desires with curiosity, not obligation.** Sharing what intrigues (or amuses) you builds intimacy before you even step into the bedroom.

3. **Explore solo.** Who says you need a partner to experiment? Many of these acts can be adapted for self-pleasure. Get creative, experiment, and learn what makes your body hum with delight.

THE BOTTOM LINE

At the end of the day, the best kind of sex is the kind where you feel seen, safe, and satisfied. So go forth, explore with enthusiasm, and remember—inner sexy is an adventure, and the map is yours to draw.

LESSON FIFTY-NINE

ONE RING TO RULE THEM ALL—WHY YOU SHOULD PUT A COCK RING ON IT

AH, the humble cock ring—an unsung hero in the symphony of pleasure. Often dismissed as mere "dick jewelry" or relegated to the nightstands of aging rock stars and overenthusiastic frat boys, this little device deserves a grander reputation. Ladies, whether you're in a long-term relationship, embarking on something new, or flying delightfully solo, the cock ring has something to offer you.

THE COCK RING CHRONICLES: A BRIEF, STIMULATING HISTORY

Long before we had medical-grade silicone and remote-controlled vibrating accessories, ancient lovers were getting creative. The Greeks, ever the connoisseurs of pleasure, were among the first to adorn their members with rings of leather and metal. But the real innovators? The Chinese. Dating back to the Jin Dynasty, men of means crafted these rings from jade, ivory, and—brace yourselves—goat eyelids (yes, with the lashes still attached). Why? Because necessity is the mother of invention, and these men needed stamina to keep up with their concubines and produce heirs.

Thankfully, modern times have delivered far more elegant

and humane options. With endless varieties—metal, silicone, vibrating, textured—there's a perfect ring for every penis (and partner) out there.

WHAT'S IN IT FOR YOU? (YES, YOU!)

So why should a woman care about cock rings? Because they're not just for him—they're for you.

- **More Time, More Pleasure** – By restricting blood flow, a cock ring helps maintain firmer, longer-lasting erections, meaning you get more time to reach your climax.
- **Hands-Free Orgasms** – Vibrating cock rings turn penetrative sex into a clitoral playground. It's like having a built-in vibrator working in tandem with every thrust—leaving your hands free to roam elsewhere.
- **Heightened Sensation** – Rings don't just delay ejaculation; they also amplify pleasure for the wearer. More sensitivity means more responsiveness, which means better chemistry for both of you.
- **Creative Play Beyond Penises** – Who said cock rings are just for cocks? Vibrating models can be placed on fingers or toys for added sensation, making them a versatile addition to any pleasure toolbox.

FINDING THE PERFECT FIT (LIKE A GOOD LOVER, IT SHOULDN'T PINCH)

Unlike shoes or lingerie, you can't exactly walk into a store and try a cock ring on for size. But don't worry—there are variety packs available, with different sizes and thicknesses to help you or your partner find the perfect fit.

- **Material Matters** – Silicone is body-safe, flexible, and easy to clean. Metal offers a firmer grip but requires precise sizing. Avoid porous materials like PVC, which can harbor bacteria. No one wants an infection.
- **Style and Function** – Some rings wrap around just the shaft; others encircle both the penis and testicles for added sensation. Vibrating models bring bonus thrills for both partners.
- **Lube Wisely** – Silicone toys require water-based lubes. Always read the manufacturer's instructions (yes, really), and, holy hell, never DIY with zip ties or carabiners—this is not a Home Depot project.

HOW TO USE ONE WITHOUT LOSING A MEMBER

A cock ring should be worn when the penis is flaccid or semi-erect, allowing the erection to grow into it—think tomato cage, but sexier. Position it either at the base of the shaft or behind the testicles for extra lift and delay.

- **Start Slow** – Begin with short sessions (five to ten minutes) and never exceed thirty unless you're aiming for an ER visit.
- **Monitor Sensation** – If there's any numbness or discomfort, remove it immediately.
- **No Overnight Stays** – Falling asleep with it on is a terrible idea—penile gangrene is not a turn-on. Yikes.

THREE TIPS TO ELEVATE YOUR RING GAME

- **Make It an Event** – Turn trying a cock ring into a playful date night experiment. Bonus points for a blindfold and a bit of mystery. You can also put one on a sex toy for my solo gals.

- **Double the Pleasure** – If you love dual stimulation, invest in a vibrating model that hits the clitoris with every thrust.
- **Beyond the Basics** – Already a fan? Upgrade to remote-controlled versions for a little public play or add a textured design for extra thrills.

THE TAKEAWAY

Cock rings aren't just for older men or performance anxiety; they're tools of pleasure, connection, and exploration. With the right fit and an open mind, they can turn good sex into great sex—whether you're playing with a partner or delighting in a little me-time. So, go ahead, put a ring on it. Your pleasure will thank you.

LESSON SIXTY

THE HOT WIFE KINK—WHEN MONOGAMY GETS A HALL PASS

Ah, mon amour, let's talk about something deliciously paradoxical: the hot wife kink. It's a scenario that flips traditional notions of monogamy, fidelity, and gender roles on their prudish little heads. The plot twist? It's often the partner who *encourages* their significant other to explore intimacy with new lovers. Intriguing, non? Let's dive in.

WHAT IS A HOT WIFE, AND WHY ISN'T SHE HOT OR A WIFE?

Much like Rhode Island, which is neither a road nor an island, the term *hot wife* is a linguistic sleight of hand. A hot wife doesn't have to be conventionally *hot* (though they certainly *feel* it), nor do they need to be legally married or even in a heteronormative relationship. What defines them is the freedom to seek out new partners—with the full encouragement (and sometimes participation) of their primary one.

But here's where things get interesting. This isn't traditional swinging, where both partners engage equally, nor is it an open relationship, where both parties date independently. Instead, hot wifing is a partner-centric exploration of pleasure. One plays, the other watches, listens, or simply revels in the knowledge that their significant other is out there living their best life. It's about desire, agency, and—perhaps paradoxically—deepening intimacy.

WHAT'S IN IT FOR THE PARTNER?

If society has conditioned us to believe partners should be territorial, why would someone *encourage* this? The reasons vary:

- **Erotic Humility** – Some people are aroused by the perceived power shift, where their traditionally "submissive" partner takes charge.
- **Compersion (Yes, That's a Word)** – Some genuinely find joy in their partner's pleasure, experiencing arousal from their satisfaction alone.
- **Arousal by Proxy** – Watching or even knowing about their partner's escapades can be intoxicating—an erotic tale unfolding just for them.

But let's be clear: this is *not* a license to philander. This isn't, "I let you, so now you let me." In a classic hot wife dynamic, the exploring partner's pleasure is the *only* priority. If the other enjoys it, it's because of *their* agency, not in spite of it.

THE FEMINIST PARADOX: SEXUAL LIBERATION OR A NEW FORM OF CONTROL?

While some hail hot wifing as the ultimate feminist expression—sexual autonomy celebrated in a traditionally heteronormative framework—it comes with caveats. If the encouraging partner is the one orchestrating every encounter, approving or rejecting lovers, and dictating the terms, then is this truly about *freedom*? Or is someone just starring in another person's fantasy?

The difference between empowerment and control lies in

intent. When both partners are equally enthusiastic, hot wifing can be an exhilarating, intimacy-enhancing experience. But if the exploring partner is merely *performing* for someone else's benefit, it risks becoming just another male-centered narrative masquerading as liberation.

Boo.

HOT WIFE VS. CUCKOLD—WHAT'S THE DIFFERENCE?

In the world of spicy dynamics, a *hot wife* is the star of the show—enthusiastically encouraged (and often *advertised*) to enjoy extracurricular activities while their partner watches, supports, or just enjoys the idea.

Meanwhile, *cuckolding* takes things a step further with a dominant/submissive twist, where the "cuck" (not always a husband, by the way) gets a thrill from being denied, teased, or even put in a more submissive role. Both kinks celebrate open exploration, trust, and—let's be honest—some seriously steamy power shifts.

Oh, and yes, hot husbands and cuckqueans are totally a thing, too.

HOW TO DO IT RIGHT: THE RULES OF THE GAME

For those intrigued by this dynamic, communication is not just a punchline—it's *paramount.*

- **Establish Boundaries Early and Often** – Define what is and isn't acceptable. Will the partner be present? Do they want details? What are the emotional and physical limits?
- **Check in Emotionally** – What feels erotic in theory can feel different in practice. Jealousy, vulnerability, or unexpected feelings may arise— talk about them.

- **Prioritize the Exploring Partner's Desire** – This is not about fulfilling *one* fantasy at the *other's* expense. The moment it stops being fun, it stops. Full stop.
- **Start with Fantasy Before Reality** – Roleplay, erotica, and guided storytelling can be sexy stepping stones before stepping into real-world scenarios.
- **Be Ready for Evolution** – What begins as a thrill might evolve into something different—or fade altogether. Keep conversations open-ended.

THE TAKEAWAY: PERMISSION, NOT POSSESSION

Hot wifing isn't for everyone, but for those who embrace it, it offers a chance to rewrite the rules of pleasure. It challenges traditional ideas of ownership in relationships and introduces a new kind of erotic play—one that hinges not on *possession*, but on *permission*. Done right, it can increase trust, communication, and intimacy. Done wrong, it can reinforce the very dynamics it claims to subvert.

So, dear reader, if you choose to explore this world, do it with curiosity, integrity, and above all—pleasure. Because the best relationships aren't about locking things down. They're about setting things free and seeing what comes back, wanting more.

LESSON SIXTY-ONE

IS THE C-SPOT YOUR PLEASURE PORTAL?

AH, my curious, pleasure-seeking souls, gather close. Today, we embark on an exploration of one of the more elusive, whispered-about frontiers of pleasure: the C-spot. Is it a mythical creature? A mapless treasure? A well-kept secret that only a lucky few have unlocked? What does the C stand for? And is three really a magic number? Let's find out.

First, a sigh of relief: this is *not* another box to check off, another milestone on the journey to self-optimization. No one is keeping score. If the C-spot is your personal nirvana, fantastic. If the mere thought of another anatomical Easter egg hunt (looking at you, Taylor Swift) exhausts you, skip it. You are no less radiant, sensual, or deserving of pleasure.

SO, WHAT EXACTLY IS THE C-SPOT?

Now the controversy begins. Some say the C stands for *clitoris*, others argue for *cervix*. But let's give the clitoris her due respect—she is not some singular *spot* but a glorious, complex, wishbone-shaped network of pleasure. If we *must* crown a singular C-spot, then let's set our gaze southward. Or inward. To the cervix.

The cervix—most commonly discussed in medical

settings, often raked during pap smears and stretched during childbirth—sits quietly at the gateway to the uterus, largely ignored in conversations about pleasure. But some cervix-owners and sex researchers claim that cervical orgasms exist, and oh, what a revelation that would be! The idea of unlocking a pleasure point so deep, so seemingly untouchable, lends the cervix an air of mystique. Oui, oui!

CERVICAL ORGASMS: MYTH, MAGIC, OR SCIENCE?

The cervix is not loaded with nerve endings like the clitoris, so how could it possibly spark orgasmic bliss? Some theories point to the *vagus nerve*—a long, wandering highway of sensation that stretches from the cervix up to the brain, bypassing the spinal cord altogether. When stimulated just right, it can trigger deep waves of sensation—more a rolling crescendo than a quick spark.

Of course, not every cervix is a pleasure portal. Some people find direct cervical stimulation uncomfortable, even painful. Timing plays a role too: during ovulation, the cervix may be more sensitive and inviting; right before a period, it might feel swollen and unapproachable. Commandment: *Know thy body, and listen to her signals.*

HOW TO EXPLORE YOUR C-SPOT

First, let's manage expectations: this is a slow, patient journey, not a bullseye to hit (trust me, if you ever wanted to know what it was like to get kicked in the balls... punch the cervix). If you want to explore, here's how to begin:

- **Start with Awareness** – Lay back, get comfy, pop on Sade's greatest hits, and pull your knees back "frog leg" style. Locate your cervix with gentle fingers. It often feels like the tip of your nose

—firm yet with some give. Take note of how it moves throughout your cycle.

- **Experiment with Containment** – Some people report that deep penetration creates a sense of fullness, of being held in a way that ignites pleasure. Try different positions, speeds, and depths to see how your body responds.
- **Use the Right Tools** – If exploring solo, longer toys with a curve can help reach the cervix without force. If exploring with a partner, communicate— slow, deep thrusts may be more pleasurable than sudden, jarring contact (again, you have my permission for a swift ball kick if that happens).

BUT WHAT IF I DON'T HAVE A CERVIX?

If you've had a hysterectomy, you may wonder, *Does this mean I can't experience deep vaginal pleasure?* Not necessarily. While some nerves are severed during surgery, pleasure is not purely anatomical—it's psychological, energetic, even mystical. The idea of *womb energy* persists in many cultures; pleasure is about sensation, yes, but also about how we relate to our bodies.

THREE TIPS FOR C-SPOT SUCCESS

- **Know Your Timing** – The cervix changes throughout the month. What's blissful one week may be uncomfortable the next. Pay attention to how your body shifts with your cycle.
- **Ease into Depth** – Cervical play is not a *thrust-and-see* situation. It requires patience, gentle touch, and—if using toys—a curve designed for precise stimulation.
- **Let Go of the Orgasm Chase** – Deep pleasure is different from clitoral pleasure. It's not about

intensity; it's about immersion. Some describe it as trance-like, slow-building, and full-bodied rather than sharp and explosive.

THE TAKEAWAY

Pleasure is personal. Whether the C-spot is your *Holy Grail* or just another letter in the alphabet of intimacy, you are still a magnificent, sensual being. Your pleasure is yours to define, discover, and revel in.

And if cervical orgasms *do* turn out to be your thing? Well then, my love, consider yourself an explorer who just mapped a new world.

LESSON SIXTY-TWO

ROCK, PAPER, SCISSORS—SCISSORING ALWAYS WINS

Let's play a little game, shall we? Rock, paper, scissors. And in this game, scissoring always wins.

Ah, scissoring—a term that makes some people giggle, others roll their eyes, and plenty more lean in just a little closer, intrigued but unsure if they should actually ask about it. Culturally, it's been both fetishized and dismissed, often misunderstood as either a joke or some mythical unicorn of queer sex. But let's set the record straight (or delightfully curved): scissoring is real, it's hot, and it's for everyone.

THE ART OF THE RUB

At its core, scissoring is a beautiful symphony of friction, a rhythmic dance of external pleasure. The name? Well, you can picture it—a delightful entanglement of legs, pelvises meeting at the fulcrum, a perfect storm of bumping, grinding, and glorious clitoral stimulation. It's a playground of pleasure, adaptable to all bodies, genders, and levels of flexibility.

It's also one of the most customizable, inclusive positions out there. People with mobility challenges? Scissoring can be adjusted to work. Height differences? Easily adaptable. And let's not forget—it's a move that prioritizes external pleasure, which, for those of us with clitorises, is a jackpot in the orgasm department.

THE MANY NAMES OF THE GAME

While *scissoring* is the pop culture darling, let's introduce a few of its relatives:

- **Tribbing:** The catch-all term for grinding one's vulva against a partner's body part (thighs, feet, face—you name it).
- **Frottage:** A French word for "rubbing," often linked to gay male culture but just as relevant to any duo seeking pleasure through friction.

Same principle, different variations. The goal remains the same: delicious, non-penetrative, body-to-body stimulation.

WHY IT'S MORE THAN JUST A POSITION

Let's be clear: scissoring is not just a 'lesbian thing'. It's not just a TikTok knee move, but naked. And it's definitely not a complex gymnastics routine requiring an Olympic-level warm-up. It's a sensual, intimate, and sometimes even playful way to connect.

What makes it special?

- **Intimacy & Eye Contact** – Unlike positions where one partner is behind the other, scissoring invites eye-gazing, synchronized breathing, and a deeper emotional connection.
- **Customization Galore** – Whether you're on your side, angled like an X, or mixing in toys and hands, it's a versatile move that allows for endless exploration.

- **A Celebration of the Clitoris** – Penetration is lovely, but let's be real: direct clitoral stimulation is often the key to the most reliable orgasms. And scissoring? It's like a VIP pass to that experience.

HOW TO GET INTO POSITION (LITERALLY & MENTALLY)

If you've seen scissoring in porn, you might think it looks exhausting—and, frankly, like a Cirque du Soleil audition. In reality, it's much simpler:

1. **Start Side by Side** – Lie down facing each other, heads at opposite ends, and start shifting those legs into position. One over, one under—wiggle, scoot, adjust.
2. **Find the Fulcrum** – The goal is to align your pelvises so that your external genitals make glorious contact. No need for aggressive thrusting; this is about rolling, rocking, and rubbing.
3. **Move with the Rhythm** – Experiment with angles, pressure, and movement until you both find a groove that works. Maybe add a pillow for support, or a little lube for glide—whatever enhances the experience.

It may take some trial and error, but sex—like all good things in life—is about the journey, not just the destination.

BUT WHAT IF IT'S . . . AWKWARD?

Spoiler alert: ooh yeah, it probably will be. You might struggle to find the right positioning. There might be a rogue queef. Someone might cramp up or pull a hamstring. And that's okay. Sex isn't meant to be a flawlessly choreographed performance—it's messy, funny, and wonderfully human.

THREE TIPS FOR WINNING AT SCISSORING

- **Pace Yourself** – This isn't a race, it's a rhythm game. Slow down, find the angles that work for *you*, and don't force a position that feels awkward or uncomfortable.
- **Add a Little Extra** – A vibrator between you, some teasing whispers, or even holding hands while moving together can heighten intimacy and pleasure.
- **Laugh It Off** – If something feels awkward, embrace it. Sex is supposed to be fun. If you both end up tangled like pretzels and laughing, you're still doing it right.

THE TAKEAWAY: SCISSOR LIKE NO ONE'S WATCHING

Scissoring isn't just a punchline—it's a deeply satisfying, playful, and intimate way to connect. So whether you're adding it to your regular rotation or just experimenting for fun, remember: when it comes to pleasure, the only rules are the ones you make.

LESSON SIXTY-THREE

SPANK YOU VERY MUCH—HOW TO SLAP SOME SASS INTO YOUR SEX LIFE

Ah, my cheeky ones, let's talk about spanking. That glorious intersection of pleasure and pain, control and surrender, dominance and delight. If the thought of a well-timed smack across the derrière sends a tingle down your spine (or straight to your pants), you are far from alone.

One survey found that over seventy-five percent of people had dabbled in BDSM. And of those? Eighty percent had experimented with spanking. And why not? Beyond the thrill of it all, spanking releases a chemical cocktail of dopamine, oxytocin, adrenaline, and endorphins, transforming a simple slap into a euphoric experience. Done right, spanking can be playful, erotic, even deeply connective. Done wrong? Well . . . let's avoid bruising anything but the ego, shall we?

A BRIEF HISTORY OF SPANKING—YOUR KINKS ARE OLDER THAN YOU THINK

Spanking for pleasure isn't new—it's ancient. Erotic spanking makes appearances in the *Kama Sutra* (circa 400 BCE), the *Koka Shastra* (1150 CE), and *The Perfumed Garden*, an Arabic guide to sensuality. The Etruscans even painted spanking scenes inside their tombs. That's commitment. By the 19th century, France and the UK had entire literary genres devoted to the subject, proving that our ancestors weren't just buttoned-up prudes—they were getting spanked in corsets and lace gloves.

So, if you've ever felt a little embarrassed about your love of a well-placed smack, remember: your great-great-grand-parents were probably into it, too.

HOW TO SPANK LIKE A PRO (A.K.A. PLEASE DON'T JUST WING IT)

If you're new to spanking, you might be tempted to just raise a hand and go for it. Don't. Spanking is an art, not a free-for-all. Here's how to do it right.

1. Set the Scene

Before any hands fly, communication is key. Ask, "Would you be into this?" rather than assuming. Establish a safe word —something short, clear, and impossible to misinterpret mid-moan (a dramatic *"KERFUFFLE!"* will work in a pinch). Discuss boundaries, intensity, and aftercare before the first smack lands.

2. Start with Your Hand

Your hand is the perfect spanking tool—it's responsive, warm, and lets you feel the impact. Start lightly, gauge reactions, and gradually build up pressure. A flat palm gives a deep, thuddy slap; fingers create a sharper sting. Mixing up sensations is where the real magic happens.

3. Find the Sweet Spots

Not all real estate is prime for spanking. The lower buttocks, the "sweet meat" (upper thighs just under the cheeks), and the outer hips are prime locations. The tailbone, lower spine, and kidneys? Off-limits unless you're trying to book a doctor's appointment instead of a second date.

4. Build Anticipation

Spanking isn't just about impact—it's about anticipation.

A slow buildup, alternating between soft caresses, teasing taps, and firm strikes, creates a delicious contrast that heightens arousal. A little breath on the back of the neck between swats? Chef's kiss.

5. Aftercare Is Mandatory

After any impact play—yes, even a casual swat—aftercare matters. This can be as simple as cuddling, massaging the warmed skin, or offering a glass of water. If bruising happens (and it might), a little arnica gel works wonders. Checking in post-play ensures trust, connection, and enthusiastic consent for next time.

TIPS FOR A SPANK-TACULAR TIME

- **Don't treat it like a punishment.** Unless explicitly agreed upon, spanking isn't about discipline—it's about pleasure. Aim for a playful, erotic tone, not a stern lecture in the principal's office.
- **Work with the rhythm.** Think build-up and release, like a drum solo, not an aggressive, out-of-sync attack.
- **Use toys to mix things up.** A paddle? A flogger? A soft leather belt? Different tools create different sensations. Experiment.
- **Know your impact.** A sharp smack leaves a sting; a broad, firm slap gives a thud. Both are hot in different ways.
- **Check in.** Mid-session "How's that feel?" is sexier than it sounds. Watching body language and listening to reactions will make you a better lover.

THE TAKEAWAY: A WELL-PLACED SPANK IS A LOVE LANGUAGE

Spanking, when done right, is playful, exhilarating, and deeply intimate. It's not about inflicting pain; it's about enhancing pleasure. It can be about surrender, dominance, power, trust, or just plain fun. But above all else, it should be consensual, communicative, and a damn good time.

So go forth, my delicious deviants, and slap responsibly.

LESSON SIXTY-FOUR

THE A-SPOT EXPEDITION: DO I NEED INDIANA JONES FOR THIS?

Ah, my curious explorers, let's embark on a sensual adventure —no dusty maps, no ancient artifacts, just a little anatomical treasure hunting. We're talking about the elusive A-Spot, a lesser-known yet potentially game-changing erogenous zone. Grab your metaphorical whip and fedora—we're going in.

THE A-SPOT: A HIDDEN GEM OR JUST ANOTHER X ON THE MAP?

If it feels like there's a new pleasure point to decode every week, you're not alone. First the G-Spot, then the C-Spot, and now the A-Spot? It sounds like we're assembling an erotic alphabet. But don't worry—I'm here to demystify this deep-spot legend and help you decide if it's worth the search.

WHAT IS THE A-SPOT ANYWAY?

The A-Spot, formally known as the **anterior fornix erogenous zone**, is nestled deep in the vagina, between the cervix and the bladder—about two inches higher than the G-Spot. Some call it the "deep spot," others lump it into the *female* *prostate* conversation. Either way, those who swear by A-Spot stimulation report it leads to:

- Deeper orgasms
- Increased vaginal lubrication
- Extended pleasure that doesn't rely on clitoral stimulation

If that last one made your eyebrows raise, you're not alone. That's reason enough to grab your explorer's hat.

IS THE A-SPOT REAL OR JUST ANOTHER EROTIC MYTH?

Unlike the G-Spot, which has been hotly debated in scientific circles for decades, the A-Spot remains a whisper in the world of sexual wellness. Most of what we know comes from a study in the late '90s, where repetitive stimulation of this area led to increased lubrication in two-thirds of participants, and 15% reached orgasm.

Not exactly conclusive, but as with all things pleasure-based, if it works for you, that's all the validation you need.

THE A-SPOT HUNT: A STEP-BY-STEP GUIDE

Picture the vagina as a soft tunnel—let's call it an under-ground pleasure cave. The A-Spot is located deeper along the **front vaginal wall**, past the G-Spot, and closer to the cervix. Here's how to find it:

1. **Start with the G-Spot:** Insert a finger and curl it upwards toward the belly button. That textured, spongy area? That's the G-Spot.
2. **Keep Going:** Move your fingers slightly deeper— about an inch or two past the G-Spot.

3. **Test for Sensitivity:** Use a slow windshield-wiper motion instead of in-and-out thrusting. If you feel pressure or warmth, congratulations, you've reached the zone.

Not feeling anything spectacular? No worries. Everyone's pleasure map is different.

TOOLS OF THE TRADE

- **Fingers:** If yours aren't long enough, a partner's might be.
- **Curved Sex Toys:** Stainless steel or borosilicate glass wands are excellent for targeted stimulation.
- **Positions:** Doggy style, lifted missionary, or anything that allows deep penetration can make the A-Spot easier to access.

WHO SHOULD CARE ABOUT THE A-SPOT?

You, if:

- You struggle with vaginal lubrication.
- You enjoy deep penetration and want to maximize sensation.
- You love a good sexual experiment and aren't afraid of a little trial and error.

HOW TO MAKE THE MOST OF THE A-SPOT EXPEDITION

1. **Approach It as a Playful Quest:** Routine is the enemy of passion. Whether solo or with a partner, treat this as a sexy adventure, not a mission to complete.

2. **Adjust Your Angle:** Deep stimulation doesn't always mean hard or fast—slow, controlled pressure is often the key to unlocking pleasure.
3. **Add Clitoral Play:** The A-Spot is powerful, but pairing it with external stimulation can take things to another level.
4. **Relax Your Pelvic Floor:** If you feel discomfort, tension might be the culprit. Deep breathing and intentional relaxation can make a huge difference.
5. **Stay Open-Minded:** If it works, fantastic! If it doesn't, that's okay—there's plenty of pleasure to be found elsewhere.

THE FINAL TREASURE: PLEASURE IS THE ADVENTURE, NOT THE ARTIFACT

Not every expedition leads to a golden idol (or an orgasmic epiphany), but that doesn't make the journey any less thrilling. Whether the A-Spot is your hidden pleasure trove or just another stop on your erotic map, the fun is in the discovery. So take your time, follow the clues, and remember—when it comes to pleasure, the adventure *is* the reward.

LESSON SIXTY-FIVE

THE LOTUS POSITION—IT WILL MAKE YOUR SEX LIFE BLOOM

Ah, my luscious lotus flowers, let's talk about a position that is as sensual as it is spiritual, as intimate as it is orgasmic, and as deeply connective as a shared bottle of Cabernet at midnight.

The Lotus—also known in Tantric traditions as *Yab-Yum*—is the ultimate invitation to slow down, sync up, and actually *be* with your partner. This isn't about frantic thrusting or breakneck acrobatics. This is about feeling, breathing, and melting into each other—body, mind, and soul.

HOW TO GET INTO THE LOTUS POSITION

Picture this: One partner sits cross-legged, comfortably grounded. The other straddles their lap, wrapping their arms and legs around them in a full-bodied embrace. Chests pressed together, lips tantalizingly close, eyes locked—or at least trying to be, before one of you gets shy and starts examining an earlobe (it happens).

The movement here is less about thrusting and more about grinding, rolling, and surrendering to the rhythm. If sex positions were cocktails, the Lotus would be a slow-sipped Negroni—complex, layered, and best savored with intention.

WHY THE LOTUS IS THE MVP OF INTIMACY

- **Eye Contact That Will Melt You**. Unlike positions where you can avoid your partner's gaze (*cough* doggy style *cough*), the Lotus requires face-to-face connection. It's vulnerable, electric, and—let's be honest—a little terrifying if you're not used to it. But lean in. This is where true intimacy starts.
- **Hands-Free Exploration**. With your hips doing the work, your hands are free to roam. Caress a back, tangle fingers in hair, tease a nipple, guide a vibrator. The Lotus is a choose-your-own-adventure playground for pleasure.
- **Perfect for Clitoral and G-Spot Stimulation**. The grinding motion and close contact make this a dream for external pleasure. Add a little lube, a well-placed pillow, or a trusty toy, and you've got a VIP ticket to Pleasure Town.

HOW TO MAKE THE MOST OF THE LOTUS

1. **Match Your Breathing**. Syncing your breaths can heighten intimacy and slow things down in the best way. Inhale together, exhale together—ride the wave of sensation.
2. **Adjust for Comfort**. If one partner has tight hips, elevate them with a cushion or try sitting on a firm surface for more support.
3. **Engage Your Core**. Rocking motions work better than thrusting here. Use your core for gentle, controlled movements.
4. **Incorporate Sensory Play**. Soft whispers, light scratching, even a silk blindfold can turn this into a full-body experience.

5. **Don't Rush the Moment**. The Lotus isn't about *finishing* fast—it's about *feeling* deeply. Savor the build-up, and if an orgasm happens, let it be a bonus, not the goal.

VARIATIONS TO KEEP THINGS INTERESTING

The Draped Lotus – The top partner leans forward, draping over their partner's shoulders for deeper penetration and G-Spot magic.

The Kneeling Lotus – Instead of sitting cross-legged, the receiving partner kneels, offering more control and a different range of motion.

The Lean-Back Lotus – Both partners lean back slightly, shifting the angle for new sensations and a different kind of delicious pressure.

FINAL THOUGHT: PLEASURE IS A JOURNEY, NOT A RACE

Trying new positions should be like trying new restaurants—sometimes you find a favorite, sometimes you just enjoy the adventure. The Lotus isn't about performance—it's about connection. So whether you find yourself entwined with a partner or on a solo escapade, take your time, breathe deep, and let pleasure unfold. Now go forth and blossom.

LESSON SIXTY-SIX

FULL SPEED AHEAD: WHY THE SPEED BUMP POSITION IS A WIN

Ah, my pleasure-seekers, let's talk about a position that deserves more hype—*The Speed Bump*. It's the perfect blend of deep sensation, full-body relaxation, and just enough effort to keep things interesting. Think of it as the *cashmere sweater* of sex positions: soft, luxurious, and always a good idea.

Unlike positions that require Cirque du Soleil-level flexibility, *The Speed Bump* is all about surrendering to pleasure without sacrificing intensity. It's perfect for lazy Sunday mornings, sultry late-night sessions, or any time you want to feel everything without doing *too much*.

HOW TO GET INTO POSITION

This one's deliciously simple: Lie on your stomach and place a pillow, bolster, or sex wedge under your hips—this is your "speed bump." Your partner kneels behind you, entering from the rear, with the elevation angling you perfectly for deep, targeted stimulation of the A, G, and C spots—the VIP lounge of internal pleasure. Rest your arms forward or tuck them beneath your body for a fully relaxed experience, or, if you want more control, push back slightly to adjust the rhythm.

WHY YOU'LL LOVE IT

- **Deep, Targeted Pleasure** – The raised hips allow for direct stimulation of high-sensation zones.
- **Effortless Bliss** – Maximum pleasure, minimum effort. No gym membership required.
- **Intimacy Upgrade** – Unlike traditional doggy style, this position allows for more skin-to-skin contact, neck kisses, and whispered confessions of just how good it feels.

SPEED BUMP PRO TIPS

Because pleasure should always be customized, here's how to fine-tune *The Speed Bump* for your body:

1. **For More Depth:** Use a firmer pillow or a taller wedge to elevate your hips even higher.
2. **For Maximum Clitoral Stimulation:** Keep a hand free for a little extra touch or introduce a small vibrator.
3. **For a Slower, More Teasing Build-Up:** Alternate between slow grinding and deeper strokes to create delicious anticipation.
4. **For Extra Control:** Bend one knee slightly outward to adjust the angle and intensity.

FINAL THOUGHT: LESS EFFORT, MORE ECSTASY

The Speed Bump is proof that good sex doesn't have to be complicated. It's intimate, indulgent, and all about savoring every sensation. So next time you want to take the express lane to pleasure, slow it down and enjoy the ride—no acrobatics required.

LESSON SIXTY-SEVEN

SWINGING 101—WELCOME TO THE PLAYGROUND

Ah, my sweet, curious pineapples—are you feeling playful today? Good. Because we're about to step onto a very different kind of playground. One that some find exhilarating, others intimidating, and many simply . . . intriguing. Let's talk about swinging: what it is, who's doing it, and, most importantly, if it might be for you.

SWINGING THROUGH THE AGES: A BRIEF, SCANDALOUS HISTORY

For most of us, the first brush with swinging likely came from pop culture—a salacious subplot in a movie, a whispered rumor about the neighbors. My first introduction? *The Ice Storm*, that '90s drama featuring a key party among 1970s suburban couples, complete with a bowl full of house keys and a lot of rum punch. At the time, I thought, *People actually do this?*

Turns out, yes. But swinging didn't start with polyester-clad suburbanites. Some trace its modern roots to the 1950s when Air Force officers in California began swapping spouses. Today, the practice has found new life in a world emboldened by the visibility of polyamory and open relationships. From private clubs in Paris to weekend retreats in suburban Florida, swinging is no longer a dirty little secret—it's just another way people explore intimacy.

WHAT SWINGING IS—AND WHAT IT ISN'T

Swinging is not polyamory. Polyamory involves deep emotional connections with multiple partners. Swinging, on the other hand, is recreational, detached, and focused on physical pleasure. It's not necessarily about seeking long-term romantic partners—it's about consensual exploration.

It's also not the same as an open relationship. Open relationships often involve independent encounters, while swinging typically happens with both partners present, in the same space (though not necessarily the same room).

WHO'S SWINGING? (HINT: IT'S PROBABLY NOT WHO YOU THINK)

Contrary to popular belief, swinging isn't just the domain of adventurous Gen Zers. It's often middle-aged couples looking to rekindle desire, urban professionals seeking a weekend thrill, and surprisingly, women are leading the charge. Gone are the days when men dragged reluctant wives along. Today, women are often the ones initiating these adventures.

THE SWINGING SPECTRUM: FROM SOFT SWAPS TO FULL SWAPS

Not all swings are created equal. Here's how the spectrum breaks down:

- **Soft Swinging** – Couples engage in sexual activity in the same room but with their own partners. Think of it as sharing the playground but staying on separate swings.

- **Full Swap** – Partners trade partners—like musical chairs, but with fewer clothes.
- **Hybrid Variations** – Some couples allow kissing and touching but not intercourse; others are open to oral but not penetration. The rules are whatever you decide.

HOW TO DIP A TOE INTO THE SWINGING POOL

1. **Start with a Conversation, Not a Proposition** – If you have a partner, approach the topic with curiosity, not pressure. "I read something interesting today . . ." is always a good opener.
2. **Explore Without Expectations** – Test the waters with books, movies, or a low-stakes visit to a swingers' club as observers. No one is making you do anything, and you can always change your mind.
3. **Understand the Etiquette** – Swinging communities thrive on respect and clear boundaries. No means no, consent is everything, and hygiene is non-negotiable.
4. **Choose Your Setting Wisely** – Swinging can happen in private gatherings, clubs, or even curated vacation resorts. Find what aligns with your comfort level.
5. **Check In—Before, During, and After** – Whether solo or with a partner, make sure the experience is meeting your needs, not just your fantasies.

THE URBAN MYTHS: PINEAPPLES, GNOMES, AND PAMPAS GRASS

Have you ever heard that an upside-down pineapple is a secret swinger signal? Or that garden gnomes, pink flamingos, and pampas grass in your yard mean you're open for business? While these may be fun urban legends, in reality, most swingers connect via apps, clubs, and word-of-mouth—not your neighbor's landscaping choices.

SWINGING SMARTER: THREE ESSENTIAL TIPS

1. **Communicate. Then Communicate Again.** If you're in a relationship, be brutally honest about your boundaries, expectations, and comfort levels. Swinging won't fix a broken relationship, but it can strengthen an already solid one.
2. **Know Your Why.** Are you swinging for self-exploration? To try something new? Because your partner wants to? Be sure you're in it for *your* pleasure, not someone else's expectations.
3. **Consent Is Sexy—And Mandatory.** Clear, enthusiastic agreement from all parties is non-negotiable. Anything less? A hard pass.

SO, SHOULD YOU SWING?

Maybe. Maybe not. The beauty of sexual exploration is that it's deeply personal. Swinging isn't a prescription for boredom, nor is it a requirement for a fulfilling sex life. It's simply an option—one more ride in the amusement park of pleasure.

If the idea makes your pulse race (in the *good* way), then why not peek over the fence and see what the fuss is about?

At the end of the day, whether you're swinging from the

chandeliers or keeping it cozy with just one, the only rules that matter are the ones you and your pleasure write together.

PART III
STRAIGHT-FROM-THE-EXPERT WISDOM

Breaking down taboos with facts, compassion, and no-nonsense advice.

LESSON SIXTY-EIGHT

FIFTY SHADES OF UNREALISTIC EXPECTATIONS: HOW TV AND MOVIES ARE MESSING WITH OUR SEXY

Ah, Hollywood. The great magician of desire. The purveyor of passion, where sex is always steamy, bodies are always flawless, and no one ever gets an ill-timed leg cramp that kills the moment. And queefs? Ha. Not even a cinematic extra.

We watch. We swoon. We wonder: Why doesn't my partner look at me and say, *"I burn for you"*? Or, *Why don't I orgasm every time I blink like Daphne Bridgerton?*

Let's get real.

THE HOLLYWOOD ILLUSION OF SEX

From *Bridgerton* to *Outlander* to *Fifty Shades of Grey*, we've been served a masterclass in cinematic seduction:

- Virginal heroines discovering earth-shattering pleasure at first thrust.
- Sex happening anywhere—against walls, on ladders, in elevators—without anyone pulling a muscle or worrying about logistics (or, God forbid, UTIs).
- Brooding men whispering sultry declarations with zero insecurity, bad breath, or second thoughts.

It's intoxicating. But it's also a lie.

Because in real life, sex is deliciously messy. Sometimes, someone's bloated. Sometimes, it's bad timing. Sometimes, one of you sneezes mid-climax. People leak. From lots of places. And you know what? That's real, and that's sexy too.

SO, WHAT'S THE PROBLEM?

The problem isn't that these stories exist—they're fun, they're fantasy, and fantasy is healthy. The issue is that they're often the only versions of sex we see. They make real intimacy feel . . . underwhelming.

If our sex lives don't look like a Netflix period drama, we wonder: Is something wrong?

No, darling. Nothing is wrong. Hollywood just skipped the part where someone asks, *"Wait, where are you putting that?"*

HOW TO RECLAIM SEXY (THE REAL KIND)

Whether you're in a long-term relationship, starting fresh, or solo and thriving, here's how to shake off the Hollywood haze and embrace real intimacy:

Rewrite the Script

- Passion isn't always spontaneous—it's curated. Plan for pleasure. A set-up can be just as sexy as spontaneity.
- Trade *"I burn for you"* for your own language of desire. Maybe it's *"I can't wait to kiss every inch of you"* or *"Let's lock the door and forget about the world."*
- Let go of the pressure for fireworks every time. Sometimes it's a slow burn, sometimes it's a flicker. Sometimes it's a dud. All are valid.

DITCH THE PERFORMANCE

- First-time sex doesn't have to be cinematic. It's okay if it's awkward, sweet, hilarious, or all of the above.
- Be honest about what you like. You're not auditioning for a role—you're co-creating a real, delicious connection.
- Don't compare your partner to fictional heartthrobs. Jamie Fraser isn't real. Your lover, with all their quirks, is. And that's infinitely hotter.

OWN YOUR NARRATIVE

- Self-pleasure isn't a sad substitute; it's a vibrant, essential part of sexuality. Explore it without shame. Be your own sexy heroine.
- Your desirability isn't measured by whether someone is pursuing you. You are sexy because you feel sexy.
- Romance yourself. Candlelit baths, lingerie, sensual touch—who says you need a partner to revel in pleasure?

THE REAL HAPPY ENDING

Hollywood sex is fantasy. Real sex is intimacy. And intimacy, in all its imperfect, awkward, deeply human glory, is where the true magic lives.

So go forth, lower your expectations, raise your pleasure, and live sexily ever after.

LESSON SIXTY-NINE

TASTE THE RAINBOW: THE WILD, COLORFUL SPECTRUM OF SEXUALITY

LET'S TALK ABOUT SEXUALITY, because it's not as clear-cut as we once thought. You've probably heard of **LGBTQ+**, but that's just the tip of the rainbow iceberg. Sexuality is fluid, ever-evolving, and deeply personal. The more we understand, the more we can respect and celebrate all the beautiful ways people experience attraction (or don't).

If you've ever felt like the standard labels don't quite fit—or if you just want to understand all the flavors on this sexual buffet—you're in the right place. Let's break down some of the most common (and some lesser-known) terms. Spoiler: this list is long (though not exhaustive), it's fascinating, and yes, it might challenge everything you thought you knew.

SEXUALITY: MORE THAN A CHECKBOX

Sexuality isn't just about gender—it's about connection, attraction, and identity. And here's the kicker: it can shift over time. Who you are today may not be who you are in ten years, and that's okay. And if you personally identify the way you always have? Fabulous. Now you can support someone else who's figuring theirs out.

While we can't list every variation (because language continues to evolve), here are some of the most common and important identities to know.

A QUICK GUIDE TO WHO'S WHO

ATTRACTION 101

- **Allosexual** – Experiences sexual attraction. (Basically, most people.)
- **Asexual** – Does not experience sexual attraction. Aces may still have romantic relationships but don't feel sexual desire.
- **Graysexual** – That in-between zone; rarely experiences sexual attraction, and when they do, it's usually mild.

THE ATTRACTION-SPECIFIC CROWD

- **Androsexual** – Attracted to masculine-presenting people (not necessarily men).
- **Gynosexual** – Attracted to feminine-presenting people (not necessarily women).
- **Demisexual** – Needs an emotional connection before experiencing sexual attraction. (No one-night stands here, darling.)
- **Sapiosexual** – Turned on by intelligence. A big brain is the ultimate aphrodisiac.

BEYOND THE BINARY: GENDER & FLUIDITY

- **Bisexual** – Attracted to more than one gender.
- **Pansexual** – Attracted to people regardless of

gender. (Not the same as bisexual, since gender doesn't factor in.)

- **Sexually Fluid** – Attraction that shifts over time or depends on the situation.

CURIOUS, EXPLORING, AND IN-BETWEEN

- **Bicurious** – Open to exploring attraction to more than one gender.
- **Heteroflexible/Homoflexible** – Mostly straight or gay but sometimes attracted to other genders.

THE "ME, MYSELF, AND I" CLUB

- **Autosexual** – Primarily sexually attracted to themselves. (No, it's not narcissism—it's self-love on another level.)
- **Sex-Repulsed** – Someone who finds the idea of sex unappealing or uncomfortable. Often falls within the asexual spectrum.

QUEER, QUESTIONING, AND EVERYTHING ELSE

- **Queer** – An umbrella term for anyone who doesn't fit neatly into heteronormative categories.
- **Questioning** – Still figuring it out. No rush, no pressure, just exploration.

WHY THIS MATTERS

Sexuality isn't black and white—it's a beautifully messy, ever-changing spectrum. Whether you find a label that fits you or just expand your understanding of the world, knowledge leads to empathy, and empathy leads to respect.

At the end of the day, that's what really matters. So, whether you're proudly skipping on the rainbow or just here for the education, remember: every identity deserves space, every person deserves acceptance, and everyone—no matter where they land—deserves to live happily, sexily ever after.

LESSON SEVENTY

CRAFTING YOUR FREEBIE FANTASY LIST—A PLAYFUL GUIDE TO UNLEASHING YOUR INNER SEXY

L ET'S TALK FANTASY LISTS. No, not the kind where you check off groceries or bills (yawn). I mean the sexy, no-strings, free-pass fantasy list—where you get to curate your dream lineup of people, places, and scenarios that ignite your inner sexy.

Because if dudes get to spend hours obsessing over fantasy football, we sure as hell get to indulge in a little fantasy fun of our own.

But this isn't just about picking Idris Elba (though, I mean . . .). This is about understanding what turns you on, why it turns you on, and how your desires evolve over time. So grab a pen (or open your Notes app), because we're about to craft the ultimate fantasy draft.

WHY MAKE A FREEBIE FANTASY LIST?

Because it's fun. Because it's revealing. Because it's a guilt-free way to explore who excites you without commitment, judgment, or needing to explain why you suddenly have a thing for that brooding villain(ess) from your latest Netflix binge.

The idea was originally born out of long-term couples who agreed that if they had an opportunity for something on the list, they were free to take it, no questions asked. But there are plenty of reasons to craft one:

- **It's a window into your desires.** The pattern of your choices—whether they're rugged, intellectual, mysterious, funny, dominant, soft, etc.—says a lot about what actually draws you in. It also shows you who else you might be open to.
- **It helps expand your fantasies.** It's not just about a *who*—it's about a *what* and *where*. Are you craving adventure? Power dynamics? A secret rendezvous in a five-star Parisian hotel? (Same.)
- **It's your permission slip for playful daydreaming.** And daydreaming, my love, is an underrated form of self-pleasure. (See Lesson Forty-Seven for a refresher on this topic!)

HOW TO BUILD YOUR FANTASY LIST

Think of this as your personal VIP guest list to your imagination's sexiest nightclub. It's not just about picking random hot people (though, respect), but curating a mix of:

- **People.** Yes, you can have Henry Cavill, but is it *him* or his Superman energy? Maybe it's the character archetype that lights your fire—the brooding protector, the charming rogue, the intellectual enigma. Maybe it's Paul Rudd's *"I never age"* endearing smirk that excites you. And perhaps . . . it's both. Put 'em on the list!
- **Places.** A moonlit beach in Greece? A swanky New York penthouse? The library from *Beauty and the Beast*? (Yes, please.) Write it on the list!
- **Scenarios.** Slow-burn romance? Power struggle? A mysterious stranger at a masquerade ball? This

is your choose-your-own-adventure. Get those adventures on the list!

WHAT "SHOULD" BE ON YOUR LIST?

Anything. You. Want.

- Celebrity crushes (but get specific—character or actor?)
- Fictional characters (Duke of Hastings, we see you)
- Daily drive-bys (that insanely hot barista who made eye contact just a second too long)
- Dreamy settings and situations (satin sheets in Santorini?)
- Moods and dynamics (do you want passion, mystery, dominance, slow-burning intensity?)

Your list, your rules. No limits. No shame. No *"but is that weird?"* (Hint: It's not.)

SHARING YOUR LIST (OR NOT)

If you have a partner, sharing lists can be hilarious, eye-opening, and oddly bonding—but only if both of you are cool about it. If they get weird and insecure, remind them that:

- **It's just a fantasy.** (You're still coming home to them and their predictable, hole-in-the-toe socks.)
- **It's a fun way to spark conversation.** (And maybe even a little inspiration.)
- **They can have their own list.** Case closed.

THE LIST EVOLVES—AND THAT'S THE FUN PART

Your freebie fantasy list isn't set in stone—it's a living, breathing, ever-changing reflection of you. What turns you on today might shift in six months, and that's normal, healthy, and hot as hell.

So write it down, revisit it, tweak it, and own it.

Now, my love—who's on your list?

LESSON SEVENTY-ONE

IS YOUR SEX LIFE ON A DIET?

Let's talk about cravings—the ones that make your mouth water, your skin tingle, and your brain light up like the Vegas strip. Food and sex. Two primal needs. Two sources of deep, undeniable pleasure. And two things women have been conditioned to feel guilty about wanting too much.

Ever notice how we talk about food the same way we talk about sex?

- Sinfully delicious
- Guilty pleasure
- Indulgent
- Forbidden fruit

Sound familiar? That's because food and sex aren't just linked—they're practically twins in the brain. In fact, the same neural pathways that drive your appetite for a juicy burger also fuel your hunger for a toe-curling orgasm.

But here's the real kicker: the way you approach food is often the way you approach sex. And if you've been stuck in an endless cycle of binging, restricting, or numbing out when it comes to eating, there's a good chance the same patterns are showing up between the sheets.

So, my love, let's pull back the covers (and maybe the fridge door) and see what's really going on.

THE SCIENCE OF CRAVING: WHY FOOD AND SEX ARE BFFS

Food and sex light up the same part of your brain—the limbic system, the OG pleasure center. This is where all the magic happens: dopamine, oxytocin, serotonin—the neurotransmitters of desire, pleasure, and bonding. When you eat something delicious, your brain throws a little party. When you have amazing sex, the same thing happens.

And just like hunger for food, sexual desire is driven by a mix of biology, psychology, and conditioning. Ever skipped a meal and suddenly found yourself ravenous and ready to devour everything in sight? That same feast-or-famine pattern can apply to sex. Deprive yourself for too long, and suddenly, you're either shutting down completely (*nope, I have a headache for the next six months*) or swinging the other way into binge territory (*hello, late-night booty call that you know damn well is a mistake*).

The brain doesn't differentiate between *"good"* pleasure and *"bad"* pleasure—it just wants the hit. And if you're not getting it one way, it'll find another route to satisfaction, whether that's polishing off a pint of ice cream, pouring another glass of wine, or scrolling through Instagram thirst traps at 1:00 a.m.

But here's the problem: we've been taught to feel guilty about pleasure. Too much food? Gluttonous. Too much sex? Slutty. And so we restrict. We suppress. We hold back.

And then we wonder why we feel so damn unsatisfied.

ARE YOU PUTTING YOUR SEX LIFE ON A DIET?

If you've ever:

- Counted calories like they were a life-or-death decision
- Labeled foods as *"good"* or *"bad"*
- Eaten a salad when you really wanted the burger
- Felt guilt after eating something decadent

. . . chances are, you've also:

- Overanalyzed your sexual desires
- Labeled certain fantasies as *"wrong"* or *"too much"*
- Had duty sex when you really wanted a toe-curling, leave-the-lights-on, breathless kind of night
- Felt guilt after an amazing orgasm (or worse, after wanting one at all)

Diet culture has trained us to see food as something to control, just like outdated sexual norms have trained us to see pleasure as something to limit. We're praised for having *"discipline"* around food, just like we're praised for not being *too much* in the bedroom. But here's the truth: just like your body needs nourishment, your sexuality needs feeding, too.

BINGE, RESTRICT, OR SAVOR? THE SEX AND FOOD CONNECTION

Let's break it down.

- **The Restrictor:** You play by the rules. No carbs after 7:00 p.m. (or, in the bedroom version: no sex unless it's scheduled and completely predictable). You don't let yourself get too hungry (or too turned on) because, well, what if you lose control? The problem? When you restrict too much, you end up feeling disconnected— disconnected from your body, your pleasure, and your partner.

- **The Binger:** You try to be *"good,"* but then—BOOM—you're elbows deep in a plate of nachos at midnight, wondering how you got there. Maybe it's food, maybe it's sex, maybe it's swiping right on someone you know isn't good for you but feels irresistible in the moment. Either way, it's a cycle of deprivation followed by overindulgence, leaving you exhausted, unsatisfied, and (let's be honest) a little regretful.

- **The Green Goddess:** Pure, clean, and in control. You thrive on discipline—whether it's organic superfoods or only engaging in *"healthy"* sex. You believe pleasure should be *earned,* and spontaneity? Not on the menu. But deep down, you want to let go—you just need permission to indulge without guilt.

- **The Junk Food Duchess:** If it's fast, fun, and gives you an instant rush—you're in. You love pleasure, no regrets! But just like a 2:00 a.m. drive-thru run, some of your choices leave you unsatisfied (or questioning your life decisions). You crave indulgence, but what would happen if you savored it instead of just consuming it?

- **The Balanced Eater (and Lover):** You eat when you're hungry, stop when you're full, and actually enjoy your food. No rules, no guilt, just listening to your body. And in the bedroom? Same deal. You let yourself experience pleasure without shame. You don't say yes when you really mean no, and you don't deny yourself what you actually crave. You understand that your appetite—whether for food or for sex—isn't something to control. It's something to honor.

FEEDING YOUR SEXUAL APPETITE—WITHOUT GUILT

- **Savor, don't restrict.** Give yourself permission to enjoy sex (yes, even the kind that isn't *goal-oriented*). Slow down. Play. Explore.
- **Indulge in variety.** No one wants to eat the same thing every night—so why are you expecting the same bedroom routine to keep you satisfied? Shake it up. Try new flavors. Expand your menu.
- **Remove the guilt.** No more labeling your desires as *"bad"* or *"too much."* You're allowed to want pleasure. You're allowed to crave it. You're allowed to feed it.
- **Listen to your body.** Are you hungry? Are you full? Are you suppressing something, or are you truly satisfied? The body always tells the truth . . . if you're willing to listen.

THE FINAL COURSE

Sex and food are both meant to be delicious. They're meant to be enjoyed, savored, and celebrated—not measured, judged, or denied.

So, my love, ask yourself: Are you letting yourself feast on pleasure? Or are you still treating it like something you have to earn?

Because the moment you stop starving yourself of what you truly desire . . .

That's when you start living (and loving) deliciously.

Bon appétit, baby.

LESSON SEVENTY-TWO

THE CONSENT COMPASS: NAVIGATING YOUR INTIMATE JOURNEY

LET'S TALK ABOUT CONSENT—NOT just as a box to check but as an ongoing conversation, a playful yet essential framework that ensures everyone's on the same page. Think of it like a GPS for pleasure: you set the route, adjust when necessary, and stay in control of the destination.

Sexual consent isn't a one-time contract; it's a living, breathing agreement that evolves as you do. Just because someone's down for a kiss doesn't mean they've signed off on everything else. And just because something felt good last time doesn't mean it's an automatic yes forever. Your desires, boundaries, and needs change—your consent should too.

KNOW YOUR GROOVE: CONSENT, BOUNDARIES, AND RULES

- **Consent** – Your enthusiastic "hell yes!" It's mutual, continuous, and revocable at any time.
- **Boundaries** – Your personal comfort zones, the non-negotiables that keep you feeling safe and respected. Example: "No unannounced paddle-room visits, please!"

- **Rules** – The hard-and-fast limits you set for yourself and others. While boundaries protect your space, rules dictate how someone else should behave. Use them sparingly—after all, intimacy should feel liberating, not like a corporate policy manual.

CONSENT CONTRACTS: NOT KILLJOYS, JUST SMART PLANNING

A consent contract isn't some rigid legal document—it's a pre-game checklist that ensures everyone's expectations align. Some critics argue that contracts take the spontaneity out of sex, but let's be real: planning your pleasure doesn't make it boring—it makes it better.

Think of it like mapping out a road trip. Sure, you might take an unexpected detour, but having a plan means you're less likely to end up somewhere you don't want to be. And here's the key: a contract isn't a binding obligation—it's a "you can unsubscribe at any time" guarantee.

THE SOBER CLAUSE: YOUR INTIMATE GPS

No one should be making big decisions while buzzed. A little wine can loosen inhibitions, but it can also blur boundaries. The sober clause ensures that every **yes** is fully informed and genuinely mutual. If you wouldn't sign a lease or make a major purchase while tipsy, why make choices about your body that way?

A Brief History Lesson. Consent has always existed in some form, but how we define it has changed drastically. In medieval times, marriages were often arranged, and a woman's consent was more about her family's honor than her personal agency. By the Age of Enlightenment, the idea of personal rights—including bodily autonomy—began to take root. Today, consent is no longer a formality; it's the foundation of healthy, empowered intimacy.

Consent Is Power, Not a Buzzkill. Some people think consent is about preventing bad experiences, but it's really about creating exceptional ones. It's about making sure no one gaslights you into compromising your boundaries. Sure, no agreement can weed out every bad actor, but when you're clear on what you want (and don't want), you're less likely to be pressured into something that doesn't feel right.

HOW TO CRAFT YOUR PERSONAL SEXUAL AGREEMENT

Whether you're in a long-term relationship or just starting to explore your sexuality, having a **personal** consent plan is like having a pleasure roadmap. Here are some ways to make it fun, functional, and fully *you*:

Set the Stage Together. Schedule a "sex strategy session"—a flirty, open-ended chat where you and your partner lay out desires, boundaries, and fantasies. Consider it a playful pre-game meeting.

Differentiate Rules vs. Boundaries. Rules are strict; boundaries are flexible. Saying, "I won't have sex unless we're exclusive" is a rule. Saying, "I don't feel comfortable with spontaneous anal play" is a boundary. Clarity is sexy.

Write It Down (Yes, Really). A mutual "intimate itinerary"—whether it's bullet points in your Notes app or an actual checklist—helps ensure expectations are clear. Think of it like updating your phone's software: revise and refresh as your needs evolve.

Plan for the Practical. Safe sex practices, a sober clause, and contingency plans (for when something unexpected happens) should all be part of the conversation. The best intimacy is built on trust, not guesswork.

USE CHECK-INS AS FOREPLAY

Consent isn't just a logistical hurdle—it can be *hot*. Try:

- **"I love the way you feel. Can I take this further?"**
- **"Tell me what you're in the mood for tonight."**
- **"What would make this experience even better for you?"**

Checking in doesn't kill the vibe—it builds anticipation.

FINAL THOUGHTS: CONSENT IS AN APHRODISIAC

Consent isn't a legal checkbox—it's a dynamic, ongoing conversation that makes sex better. It's the mutual, enthusiastic green light that keeps the vibe flowing.

Your sexual agreement isn't a contract—it's a roadmap to pleasure. Revise it, tweak it, and let it evolve with you. It's not about restrictions; it's about freedom. Because the sexiest thing you can bring into the bedroom—besides that killer lingerie— is absolute clarity in what you want.

Now go forth, explore, and navigate your pleasure with bold, unapologetic confidence.

LESSON SEVENTY-THREE

HOW TO KEEP YOUR LADY GARDEN HAPPY AND HEALTHY

HELLO, darling. Are you feeling *vulvicious* today? Yes, I made up that word—because your vulva deserves to be celebrated, pampered, and properly cared for.

Think of your genitals like a delicate houseplant—thriving with the right balance of hydration, airflow, and gentle attention. But unlike my doomed angel-wing cactus (RIP), your lady garden has built-in self-maintenance. You just need to support her natural ecosystem.

SEASONAL CARE FOR YOUR SOUTHERN HEMISPHERE

Winter doesn't *dry out* your vagina—that's a myth. But your vulva? That's another story. Cold weather, tight yoga pants, sweaty swimsuits, and whatever was in that holiday gift basket from your office Secret Santa (*please step away from the glitter lotion*) can leave her cranky and irritated.

One patient learned this the hard way after an allergic reaction to her very own sparkle party. Shimmering hives? Not sexy.

HOW TO TEND YOUR GARDEN LIKE A PRO

- **Wash Wisely** – Your vulva isn't a nightclub; she doesn't need to smell like *Midnight Reverie en Paris.* Stick with a neutral pH wash or plain water.
- **Moisturize Mindfully** – A dab of olive oil, bio oil, or Aquaphor can soothe dry spells. Crisco (yes, **that** Crisco) if you're truly feeling daring.
- **Trim Thoughtfully** – Use a gentle trimmer, not a weed whacker. Pubic hair curls naturally, so shaving too close can cause ingrowns, and ingrowns can turn into abscesses. Also, if you borrow your partner's beard trimmer... . . . *please* disinfect it first.

PH, PERIODS, AND PLAYTIME

Your vagina is a chemistry queen with a naturally acidic pH to fend off infections. What throws her off balance? Semen, period blood, and overzealous cleaning. So skip the douches (literally and metaphorically)—your vagina is a masterpiece, not a DIY home reno project.

If something smells off, **call your provider, not Dr. Google.**

LOVING YOUR LADY BITS: TIPS FOR EVERY SITUATION

- **For long-term lovers:** Introduce a sensual self-care ritual together. A gentle vulva massage with a nourishing oil? Intimacy and wellness in one.
- **For new romances:** Confidence and honesty in bed matter more than chemistry. If someone pulls out a new *strawberry-flavored glitter lube*, politely decline on behalf of your labia.

- **For self-care queens:** Make self-checks and self-pleasure part of your routine. You're the CEO of your **pleasure portfolio**—own it.

So here's to living sexily ever after—soft, smooth, and sparkly where it counts . . . *irritation-free!*

LESSON SEVENTY-FOUR

WHEN PEE PLAYS HARD TO GET—AND HARDER TO HOLD

Ah, my curious kitten, today we step into a subject that's more puddle than passion: urinary incontinence. Not the sexiest of topics, I know—but trust me, the ability to sneeze without surprise is a cornerstone of living sexily ever after. Because when you're worried about leaks, it's hard to feel luscious between the sheets (and you can quote me on that!).

THE UNSEEN INTRUDER: INCONTINENCE IN MIDLIFE

Maybe you're thinking, *I'm thirty-eight. I don't have incontinence. Why are we here?* Well, darling, urinary leaks don't RSVP before they arrive. Nearly 20 percent of adults over eighteen wrestle with an overactive bladder, and by forty, it's one in five. The stats only climb as we age. Incontinence, much like desire, is democratic—it doesn't care about your age, relationship status, or the hotness of your lingerie.

So let's demystify this bladder rebellion. There are two headliners here:

Urge Incontinence (The "Gotta-Go-Now" Frenzy) – Ever feel like the bathroom is a ticking time bomb? If you can't hold it once the signal hits, you may be dealing with an overactive bladder. It's the real-life version of that old commercial jingle: *Gotta go, gotta go, gotta go right now.*

Stress Incontinence (The Surprise Spritz) – Laugh, sneeze, cough—and whoop, there it is. If you've ever crossed your legs mid-sneeze like a pelvic-floor ninja, you're not alone. It happens when pressure overpowers a weakened urethra, like a muscle that's lost its edge.

And here's a personal confession: Once, during a robust coughing fit, I peed so forcefully it hit my pants like a rogue water pistol. The wet spot? Right at knee level. I strutted out of the bathroom, casually flicking water on my pants to pass it off as a faucet mishap. Shame? Please—I choose humor over humiliation every time.

WHY PEE MATTERS FOR PASSION

Incontinence messes with your mind. It's tough to enjoy naked intimacy when you're secretly praying your bladder doesn't stage a coup. But here's the truth: addressing the issue isn't just about convenience; it's about confidence. And confidence, my love, is the ultimate aphrodisiac.

THREE TIPS FOR SEXY, SECURE BLADDERS

1. **Laugh About It** – Humor neutralizes shame. If you sprinkle mid-laugh, own it with a giggle. Vulnerability can spark intimacy—and a bathroom break can become part of the story.
2. **Pelvic Playtime** – Strengthen that pelvic floor with regular Kegels or, better yet, pelvic floor physical therapy. In France, new moms get it as standard care. Why? Because strong pelvic muscles equal better bladder control *and* better orgasms. *Oui, oui.*

3. **Bathroom Pre-Game** – Make "just-in-case" bathroom visits part of foreplay. It's practical, playful, and sets the stage for carefree intimacy.

Pro Tip: Worried about eau de pee? A light dusting of cornstarch in your underwear works like a charm—absorbing odor faster than you can say *whoops*. Bonus: it keeps things fresh without turning your lady bits into a perfume counter.

FINAL SPLASH: OWN YOUR FLOW

Incontinence might feel like an unexpected plot twist, but it's hardly the end of your sexy story. Your body isn't betraying you—it's just asking for a little extra TLC. With the right tricks (and a good sense of humor), you can sneeze, laugh, and orgasm without a second thought. So go forth, stay fabulous, and let confidence—not your bladder—take the lead.

LESSON SEVENTY-FIVE

THE PLEASURE MAP: UNLOCKING YOUR EROGENOUS ZONES

WE'RE DIVING into the fascinating, often overlooked terrain of your erogenous zones—the secret pleasure map of your body. You might think you already know the highlights, but trust me, there's more to explore. And yes, we're doing this for science (but mostly for fun).

YOUR BODY'S HIDDEN PLEASURE CENTERS

Monica from *Friends* once famously schooled the guys on the seven female erogenous zones, building up an orgasmic crescendo like a conductor orchestrating a symphony. The truth? There are way more than seven. And when it comes to pleasure, skipping the warm-up is like going to the Grand Canyon and only seeing the parking lot.

According to research, the top five erogenous zones (in descending order) are: breasts, lips, neck, ears, and butt. But that's just the beginning. Let's take a sensual tour, shall we?

THE SCIENCE OF SENSATION

Your body is brimming with nerve endings beyond the usual pleasure zones, and studies show that over 10 percent of women can orgasm purely from stimulating extra-genital areas. So if you haven't explored beyond the usual suspects, consider this your invitation.

Erogenous Zones to Explore

1. **Ears** – The nerve endings here are plentiful, which is why whispering, nibbling, or even just warm breath can be wildly arousing. Run your fingers over the outer ear, gently massage the lobe, or let your partner trace it with their tongue. Bonus points for a slow, hushed whisper of something delicious.
2. **Nape of the Neck** – This classic hotspot is made for gentle kisses, teasing fingertips, and slow, deliberate breaths. There's a reason why the term *necking* exists—it works.
3. **Lower Back** – Often ignored, the lower back is tension-filled and nerve-rich. Try slow caresses, firm massages, or light scratches trailing up and down the spine.
4. **Inner Wrists** – The thin skin and pulse points make this an unexpectedly erotic place. A lingering touch, a featherlight kiss, or the warmth of a mouth hovering just above? Shiver-inducing.
5. **Fingertips** – Your fingers are packed with sensitive nerve endings. Ever had someone lightly suck or kiss your fingertips? Try it. It's intimate, sensual, and incredibly underrated.
6. **The Happy Trail** – The soft skin from your belly button downward is ultra-sensitive, making it perfect for slow, teasing touches or warm palm pressure. A trail leading to adventure, if you will.
7. **Armpits** – Yes, really. They contain pheromones that trigger attraction and can be surprisingly sensual when kissed, touched, or lightly stroked. Just make sure the ticklish factor is in check.

8. **Behind the Knees & Inner Elbows** – These rarely touched areas have thin, nerve-dense skin. A soft caress or playful nuzzle can send unexpected waves of pleasure through your whole body.

THREE WAYS TO INTEGRATE THIS INTO YOUR LOVE LIFE

Rediscover Each Other – Create a pleasure map. Set aside time to explore every inch of each other's skin, discovering which areas spark the strongest reactions. No rush, no agenda —just curiosity.

Turn Foreplay into a Treasure Hunt – Instead of diving straight into the usual routine, spend extra time on these zones. Make it playful, exploring with fingertips, lips, and teasing touches to see what builds the most anticipation.

Make Self-Discovery a Ritual – Your pleasure is yours to explore. Use warm oil, soft fabrics, or even a feather to trace your own skin. Pay attention to what feels unexpectedly good. The more you know, the more you can enjoy—alone or with a partner.

YOUR NEW MANTRA

Repeat after me: My body is a treasure map of pleasure, and I give myself permission to explore every inch of it.

THE BOTTOM LINE

Sexuality is about presence, play, and possibility. Whether you're with a partner or on a solo expedition, let yourself delight in all the pleasure your body has to offer. Because, darling, you are absolutely *zoned* for it.

LESSON SEVENTY-SIX

THE SYMPHONY OF YOUR BODY—WHY FARTS, BURPS, AND QUEEFS

SHOULDN'T KILL THE MOOD

Ah, the human body. So exquisitely designed for pleasure, yet so capable of surprise sound effects. One moment, you're a sensual goddess, moaning in ecstasy, and the next—your body releases an unexpected encore. A burp, a queef, a fart—the great equalizers of intimacy.

But here's the thing: desire doesn't thrive in a vacuum of perfection. If we wait for the moment when our bodies make no noise, our hair stays gravity-defying, and our stomachs never bloat, we'll be waiting forever.

WHY ARE WE SO EMBARRASSED?

From the moment we hit puberty, we were sold the idea that "feminine" means composed, pristine, and rose-scented. Meanwhile, men are socially permitted—nay, encouraged—to belch with abandon, slap their beer bellies, and turn bodily functions into competitive sports.

But here's the truth: the ability to be uninhibited is sexy. The ability to laugh when our bodies do what bodies do is a turn-on. Science backs this up—humor ranks in the top five most desirable traits in long-term relationships. If you can laugh in the bedroom, you can laugh through life. And isn't that what makes a connection last?

SCIENCE SAYS: YOUR BODY IS A WIND INSTRUMENT

Let's get clinical for a moment.

- Queefs (vaginal flatulence): The poetic term for air getting trapped and then released from the vagina, often in acrobatic positions. Not a digestive function, just physics.
- Burps (eructation): The body's way of releasing swallowed air. Nervous? Giggling? Moaning a little extra? Voilà—welcome to aerophagia.
- Farts (flatus): Gas happens. And when sex positions involve hip elevation or deep penetration, well, let's just say the pressure has to escape from some hole.

So what's a lady to do when nature calls at the most inconvenient moment? Lean in. Own it. Make it part of the experience, rather than the end of it.

THREE TIPS FOR HANDLING 'ERUPTIONS' LIKE A SEX GODDESS

1. **Rewrite the script.** Call it *bedroom jazz*, declare yourself a *saxophone of seduction*, or just grin and say, "Guess my body wanted a standing ovation." Humor diffuses awkwardness before it can take root.
2. **Smirk, don't shrink.** New relationships tempt us to act like airbrushed, noise-free versions of ourselves, but sexy isn't silent. Instead of freezing

in horror, own it with a smirk: "Congratulations, you just unlocked a secret level." The right partner won't flinch. Confidence is hotter than perfection.

3. **Radical self-acceptance, baby.** Ever burp alone and still say "Excuse me" to an empty room? Ask yourself—who are you apologizing to? Treat every unexpected sound like a stretch or a sigh— because that's all it is.

YOUR NEW MANTRA

Repeat after me: I am not a porcelain doll. I am a living, breathing, pleasure-seeking being. My body is a vessel of desire, and if it sings along the way, so be it.

Let go of the idea that sex must be poised, perfect, and immaculate. Let your body move, moan, and make music. The right people? They'll love the soundtrack.

LESSON SEVENTY-SEVEN

NIP SLIPS AND PLEASURE TRIPS: THE NIPPLE FACTS EVERYONE NEEDS TO KNOW

Ah, nipples—tiny but mighty, often overlooked yet packed with power. They perk up when we're cold, disappear when we least expect it, and occasionally make unexpected red carpet appearances. But beyond wardrobe malfunctions and the breastfeeding gig, nipples are sensual superstars, brimming with untapped pleasure.

So let's get up close and personal with these underestimated gems because, darling, they deserve their moment in the spotlight.

THE NIPPLE: A TINY (YET MIGHTY) PLEASURE HUB

Nipples are one of the few erogenous zones that all genders share, meaning pleasure isn't just a "down south" experience. Whether they're flat, perky, inverted, or somewhere in between, all variations are completely normal—think sisters, not twins. And yes, some people are blessed with extra (supernumerary) nipples. Even Mark Wahlberg reportedly has a bonus one. (No word on whether it has its own acting career.)

And let's not forget the areola—the ring around the nipple that's basically the VIP lounge of sensation. It can darken, change size, and yes, even grow a rogue hair or two (totally normal, and no, you're not turning into Sasquatch).

NIPPLES & THE BRAIN: A DIRECT PLEASURE LINE

Here's a fun fact to toss out at your next dinner party: nipple stimulation lights up the same brain regions as genital stimulation. That's right—your brain can't tell the difference between an orgasm from below and one that's all about the nips. And for some lucky souls, nipple stimulation alone can trigger an orgasm (known as a "nipplegasm" and unofficially known as proof that the body is a freaking wonderland).

Cold weather, excitement, arousal? The blood vessels in your nipples contract, making them stand at attention—your very own pleasure barometer.

THREE WAYS TO CELEBRATE YOUR NIPPLES

The Nipple-Only Foreplay Challenge

Long-term lovers, let's be real—sometimes we rush to the finish line, skipping all the delicious build-up. Time to switch things up. Dedicate twenty minutes to nipple exploration only —no jumping ahead. Experiment with:

- Ice cubes (a shivery thrill)
- Feathers (sensory teasing)
- Light sucking (tried & true)
- Nipple clamps (if you're feeling bold—but please, no chip clips or DIY garage equipment)

The goal? Anticipation. See how long you can make the tension last.

The Nipple Whisperer Challenge

Here's a fun way to test the waters with a new partner— take turns exploring each other's nipples with different touches:

- Soft flicks
- Circular motions
- Gentle biting

Rate each sensation from one to ten (because communication is sexy). You'll quickly discover what sends sparks flying—and maybe pick up a few new tricks along the way.

Unlock the Power of the Nipplegasm

While the nipple has one-tenth the nerve endings of the clitoris (800 vs. 8,000), women *can* reach orgasm from nipple stimulation alone—and if that's not self-love goals, I don't know what is.

Try:

- Light pinching or rolling between your fingers
- Brushing a silk scarf over them
- Using a vibrator (game-changer, trust me)

THE BOTTOM LINE

Your body is capable of some pretty wild things—why not see what it can do?

Whether in erotica or real life, nipples are far too often ignored, rushed, or treated as a warm-up act—but they can be a headliner (or headlights) all on their own. Let's stop treating them like an afterthought and start celebrating them for the pleasure powerhouses they truly are.

So go forth, darlings—flick, tease, and give those nips the standing ovation they deserve.

LESSON SEVENTY-EIGHT

THE ART OF THE SQUEEZE: WHY KEGELS SHOULD BE YOUR MAIN SQUEEZE

Let's parlay about something that deserves far more attention than it gets—your pelvic floor. More specifically, the great and powerful Kegel. These tiny contractions are the unsung heroes of bladder control, strong orgasms, and keeping everything exactly where it's supposed to be. They are also wildly misunderstood, underutilized, and, let's be honest, not exactly the sexiest exercise in the repertoire. Until now.

WHY SHOULD YOU CARE?

Because your vagina is a freakin' masterpiece. It is, as one wise woman once described, like an orange juice can—cylindrical, flexible, and capable of expanding and contracting as needed. The trouble is, as we mature, we start to lose the collagen that once kept everything bouncy, supple, and, yes, delightfully wrinkly (and in her case, wrinkles are a good thing!). Without a little maintenance, things can start to feel . . . let's call it unmoored.

KEGELS: WHAT YOU NEED TO KNOW

First of all, let's get the pronunciation straight. It's Kegel, like bagel, not Kegel, like beagle. And it's essentially vaginal yoga —or *Voga*, if you will (I'm making this a thing). The problem? Most women don't know how to do them correctly, or at all. They either squeeze the wrong muscles or go overboard, treating Kegels like an Olympic event and ending up with a pelvic floor strain. Not sexy.

So how do you know you're doing them right? Let's set the scene.

THE ELEVATOR TEST (AKA, HOW TO IDENTIFY YOUR KEGEL MUSCLES)

Imagine you're in an elevator, heading to the 26th floor. You're alone—until the doors open, and in walks your ultimate fantasy celebrity crush (this can also be the hottie from the local coffee shop). You exchange a polite, yet slightly smoldering glance. And then (cue cinematic disaster movie music) . . . your stomach rumbles. The five-alarm chili you had last night wants revenge.

You feel something is about to escape. We're at DEFCON 2 with IBS causing a sweaty, fight-or-flight gurgling of the guts. But you clench every muscle down there to avoid a **sh*taster**. You suck *up* every hole—your bladder, your vagina, your rectum—because under no circumstances will you become the woman who explosively sharts in front of Henry Cavill. (*Oh, and don't forget to breathe.*)

And . . . *scene*. That, my dear, is a proper Kegel. Honestly, I'm spent.

HOW TO MAKE KEGELS A HABIT

Now that you know what to do, the question is when to do it. Here's a plan that fits effortlessly into your daily routine.

The Silent Kegel Pact

Have a secret Kegel signal between you and a trusted friend or partner—like a certain phrase or a playful tap—so when one of you does a squeeze in public, the other knows and joins in. It's your sexy little inside joke, and it makes even the most boring moments more fun.

Try doing Kegels while watching a comedy special or sharing funny stories. Laughing naturally engages the pelvic floor, making it a lighthearted way to train your muscles. (*Let's be real—laughing during Kegel training is a core memory in the making.*)

Sneaky Stoplight Workouts

Every traffic signal is an opportunity for pelvic floor greatness. At a red light, squeeze and lift for five seconds, release, repeat. Two or three rounds before the light turns green, and boom—your Kegels are done for the day. Bonus: Give the driver next to you a mischievous glance and perhaps a cheeky wave. They have no idea you're strengthening your orgasm game at that very moment.

The Bedroom Bonus Round

Want to know a little secret? Kegels during sex = game-changer. Try a few mid-action, and I promise you, someone—likely you—will *definitely* notice.

THE BOTTOM LINE

Kegels are your ticket to pleasure, confidence, and pelvic health. And the best part? Henry Cavill never needs to know.

LESSON SEVENTY-NINE

TABOO-TAY! HERE'S WHAT YOU NEED TO KNOW ABOUT ANAL SEX (BUTT FEEL TOO AWKWARD TO ASK!)

LET'S TALK ABOUT BUTTS, baby. Specifically, the fact that everyone has one—and yet, anal sex remains one of the most taboo, whispered-about, and (frankly) misunderstood aspects of sexual exploration.

Some people are curious about it. Some love it. Some are completely grossed out by the idea. And hey, all reactions are valid. But here's the thing: anal sex isn't new (history proves that), and it's not as simple as porn makes it look. So if it's on your radar (or your partner's wishlist), let's get into the nitty-gritty—because this is one sexual experience where a little knowledge can make all the difference.

FIRST THINGS FIRST: THE SCIENCE OF THAT BACKDOOR BUSINESS

A quick anatomy refresher:

- **The anus:** The external opening, home to a lot of nerve endings.
- **The rectum:** The internal canal just beyond the anus.

- **Sphincter muscles:** The gatekeepers of anal entry and the reason why forceful, unprepared penetration is a big no-no (it's like shoving a barge through a drinking straw).
- **Nerve central:** The pudendal, perineal, and pelvic nerves all hang out here, meaning stimulation can feel really, really good—or really, really bad if done wrong.

And the most important lesson of all?

The anus does NOT self-lubricate.

Unlike the vagina, it produces zero moisture. So without lube, you're basically sandpapering your way to pain, tears, and possibly an ER visit.

THE BIG QUESTIONS (AND MY HONEST, DOCTOR-BASED ANSWERS)

Will anal sex make me poop my pants?

No, your rectum won't just give out in the middle of Trader Joe's. Just like the vagina after childbirth, the anus is designed to stretch and return to normal. But if you have pre-existing pelvic floor issues, heavy anal play could contribute to weakness—so, Kegels are your friend.

Will anal sex mess with my hemorrhoids?

If you've got hemorrhoids the size of a small city, inserting anything is going to be uncomfortable. Avoid sticking anything up there until they're healed, and when you do try, use a thick, creamy lube (yes, the kind gay men have been perfecting for decades).

Can I get an STI from anal sex?

1000% yes. Gonorrhea, chlamydia, herpes, syphilis, HPV, HIV—you name it, it can live back there. Using condoms and getting tested is essential.

And for the love of all things sanitary:

NO DOUBLE DIPPING.

- Vagina first, anus second? Sure.
- Anus first, vagina second? Hell. No.

What if there's poop?

It happens. If you're engaging in anal play, accept the reality that your partner may encounter some surprises. Many people prep with enemas or high-fiber diets beforehand. And if something happens? Laugh it off, clean up, and move on.

Why do some women like anal sex?

- Nerve endings make it pleasurable (it's basically an orgasmic goldmine).
- Pressure from penetration can feel amazing on the vaginal wall.
- It's a little "forbidden"—and that can make it hot.
- It makes their partner happy (though this should NEVER be the only reason to do it).

So Should I Try It?

That depends on YOU. If you're genuinely curious—great. If you're doing it just to please your partner—pause. The best anal experiences happen when you:

- Feel completely in control
- Have mutual trust with your partner
- Use lube, lube, and more lube
- Communicate every step of the way

Dr. B's PSA: If It Goes In, It Needs A Base!

WARNING: The rectum loves to suck things up and never return them. I've seen everything from light bulbs to Hot Wheels to literal vegetables make their way into ER reports. So if you're exploring toys—make sure they have a flared base. Otherwise, you may end up explaining your life choices to a very amused surgeon.

FINAL THOUGHTS: TO TRY OR NOT TO TRY?

At the end of the day, anal sex isn't mandatory, but neither is it shameful. Some people love it, some people don't, and that's okay. The key is understanding your own desires, communicating openly, and NEVER feeling pressured to do something that doesn't feel right.

So whether you're just curious, ready to go, or still clutching your pearls—just remember: your body, your rules, your pleasure. And always, always honor thy asshole.

LESSON EIGHTY

NIP AND TUCK FOR YOUR LADY BITS—WHY GENITAL COSMETIC SURGERY IS ON THE RISE

FEELING PARTICULARLY AESTHETIC TODAY? Let's talk about something that's growing in popularity but rarely discussed with the honesty it deserves—genital cosmetic surgery.

You've probably stood in front of a mirror, squinting, twisting, tilting, thinking: *Is everything symmetrical down there?* Maybe you've had an unfortunate moment with a handheld mirror and a tiled bathroom floor. Maybe you do a lot of hot yoga and can look without a mirror. And maybe—just maybe—you've wondered if your partner secretly harbors an opinion about your uniquely beautiful genitals.

Let's be clear: there is no standard-issue vulva. Shapes, sizes, and colors vary widely, and—fun fact—half of all women naturally have labia minora that extend beyond the majora. And yet, the desire to tweak, trim, or tighten continues to rise. Between 2014 and 2018 alone, female genital cosmetic surgery procedures increased by more than 50 percent. Why?

THE TOP THREE REASONS WOMEN OPT FOR GENITAL COSMETIC SURGERY

1. **The Brazilian Effect.** Once upon a time, pubic hair concealed everything. Then came the reign of waxing, shaving, and laser hair removal. When the curtains went up, some women became hyper-aware of what was previously unseen. And like any other body part exposed to scrutiny, insecurities followed.

2. **The Internet and Unrealistic Comparisons.** From porn to OnlyFans, the vulvas we see online tend to be curated, surgically altered, or simply filtered. If your primary exposure to other women's bodies comes from these sources, you might start thinking something's *wrong* with yours. Spoiler alert: there's not.

3. **It's Not Just for the Cosmo Crowd.** Surprise! Women over forty-five are more likely to consider cosmetic genital surgery than their younger counterparts. Why? Aging changes everything—skin loses elasticity, the vulva loses its youthful fullness, and gravity does what gravity does. For some, a little surgical intervention feels like reclaiming youth and confidence.

THE MOST COMMON PROCEDURES (AND WHAT YOU SHOULD KNOW)

- **Labiaplasty.** Reduces the length of the labia minora, often to prevent twisting, tugging, or just for aesthetic preference. It's the most commonly performed genital cosmetic procedure.

- **Clitoral Hood Reduction.** Removes excess folds

around the clitoris to create a more *balanced* look and let Hedwig peek out her angry inch.

- **Labia Majora Augmentation or Reduction.** Either trimming excess skin or adding volume via fat transfer (or sometimes filler).
- **Monsplasty.** A *tummy tuck* for the pubic mound, often requested post-C-section.
- **Vaginoplasty.** Tightens the circumference of the vaginal canal, usually sought after post-childbirth or due to aging.

THE REAL TALK: SHOULD YOU DO IT?

Plastic surgery can be empowering, but it should never be driven by shame or an unrealistic beauty standard. And if your partner is pushing you toward it? Let me be blunt: dump their ass. If they're that concerned with aesthetics, they can book their own scrotal lift first (which is an actual procedure . . . seriously . . . YouTube it!).

THREE SEXY, SMART ALTERNATIVES TO SURGERY

1. **Pelvic Floor Play.** A sleeker, more responsive vagina isn't just about surgery—Kegels, resistance training (yes, vaginal weights exist, though I don't recommend trying to lift a surfboard with your clam), and pelvic floor physical therapy can work wonders. Plus, they enhance orgasms. Win-win.
2. **Confidence Rituals.** Instead of scrutinizing your vulva, celebrate it. Practice mirror affirmations (*I am uniquely beautiful*), invest in soft, sensual lingerie, or take boudoir photos that make you feel like the goddess you are. As the Kardashians taught me about selfies: it's all about angles. Make sure any 'vulvies' that you take

(vulvar selfies, this WILL catch on) have proper lighting and angles to check out your own junk.

3. **Pleasure First.** Before considering surgery, explore what truly feels good. Cutting tissue can change the nerve endings in your genitals. Self-pleasure with different sensations—temperature play, feather-light touch, or vibration—can teach you to love and appreciate your body in all its natural glory.

YOUR NEW MANTRA

My body is a masterpiece, sculpted by time, experience, and pleasure. I am already enough.

THE BOTTOM LINE

If you choose to tweak the masterpiece, make sure it's for the artist—you. Because, my gorgeous, perfection was never the goal—power, pleasure, and self-love are.

LESSON EIGHTY-ONE

BRAVE AND UNASHAMED—REWRITING THE HERPES NARRATIVE FROM STIGMA TO STRENGTH

Hello, my radiant rebel. Welcome to another lesson in living sexily ever after. Today, we're tackling a topic that calls for a gigantic burst of courage: genital herpes. Yes, that virus often shrouded in stigma like a big scarlet "H." But here's the revelation—bravery, radical self-acceptance, and unfiltered honesty are the most alluring forms of intimacy. Embracing your whole self, herpes and all, isn't just liberating—it's downright sexy.

UNDERSTANDING THE SITUATION

Herpes isn't a verdict; it's simply part of the human experience. More than 20 percent of the world's adult population carries it—often unknowingly—and it doesn't diminish your beauty or desirability. There are two main players:

1. **HSV-1** – Known for cold sores (and sometimes, yes, appearing on the genitals). More than 60 percent of the world's population has this virus.
2. **HSV-2** – The form most often linked to genital outbreaks (more than 850 million people—or more than ten percent—across the globe carry this form).

While outbreaks can feel challenging—with flu-like symptoms and painful sores—they're simply moments in your body's ongoing conversation with a common virus. With modern antiviral treatments, consistent self-care, and the courage to communicate openly, you can live a passionate, fulfilling sex life—free of shame and stigma.

THE ART OF SELF-CARE AND RADICAL HONESTY

First and foremost, treat your body with the kindness it deserves. When an outbreak occurs, give yourself permission to rest and heal. Some self-care practices include:

Soothing Remedies – Enjoy warm baths with Epsom salts, apply doctor-recommended creams, and even skip underwear when needed for extra relief.

Medication – Adhere to your antiviral regimen to help your body manage the virus and speed recovery.

Creative Intimacy – Remember, connection isn't limited to intercourse. Explore sensual massages, mutual self-exploration, or simply share cuddles that nurture both body and soul.

And now, let's celebrate the transformative power of honesty. Telling someone about your herpes status is not a moment of vulnerability to hide behind—it's a testament to your bravery and the deep intimacy you're willing to build. Choose a calm, private moment to share your truth. You are not dirty. You are not tainted. Your honesty invites a deeper connection, showing that you value transparency and care about your partner's well-being as much as your own.

THREE SMART, SEXY STRATEGIES FOR NAVIGATING HERPES WITH CONFIDENCE

1. **Develop a "Bravery Pact".** Whether in a relationship or dating, create a personal

understanding that honest communication is your superpower (I mean, the ability to fly is soooo basic). Agree on ways to talk about sexual health—not as a barrier, but as an act of care.

2. **Keep It Brief, Bold, and Beautiful.** Herpes is common, manageable, and not a reflection of your worth. Have a prepared, confident explanation ready: "I have herpes—a common part of life that I manage responsibly. It's just one aspect of who I am, and I'm proud of my honesty." A touch of humor can smooth the way.

3. **Promote Mutual Empowerment.** Sexual health is a two-way street. Invite your partner to share their own experiences. Mutual testing and transparency are stepping stones to building a strong, trusting foundation.

THE TAKEAWAY

Herpes might be a part of your story, but it doesn't define your narrative. Every twist in life is an opportunity to embody courage, authenticity, and passion. Radical self-acceptance and honest communication are the ultimate acts of intimacy —both with yourself and with others.

So live boldly, speak your truth, and never let anyone dim your inner flame. Keep it sexy, keep it honest—and, as always, keep it yours.

LESSON EIGHTY-TWO

HPV UNMASKED—NAVIGATING THE NASTY WITH CONFIDENCE AND CONNECTION

WELCOME to another candid lesson in living sexily ever after. Today, we're diving into the world of human papillomavirus (HPV)—that notorious, sneaky little virus that's as common as it is misunderstood. Before you recoil, let's get one thing straight: almost everyone will encounter HPV at some point, and it's not a reflection of your character or your sexual prowess. In fact, it's just one more twist in the beautiful, messy dance of human intimacy.

THE SKINNY ON HPV

HPV is the ghosting ex of the viral world—it shows up unannounced, lingers unpredictably, and sometimes disappears without a trace. Around 80 percent of us will be exposed at least once. It's not just about cervical cancer (which, yes, is serious) but also a host of other issues like genital warts, anal, penile, and even mouth and throat cancers. HPV loves to hang out at the intersection of skin and mucosa—those glistening, delicate borders that we often take for granted. It doesn't discriminate: whether you're in a committed relationship, casually dating, or simply minding your own business, HPV can touch all of our lives.

Now, here's the real talk: there's no cure for HPV, but there's plenty we can do to manage it. Prevention, early detection, and open communication are your best allies. And yes, there's a vaccine that's recommended for both boys and girls —so get on board, no matter your age (up to forty-five, as it stands).

TALKING ABOUT HPV: THE ART OF RADICAL TRANSPARENCY

When it comes to sharing your HPV status, timing is everything. Choose a quiet moment—perhaps over coffee, during a chill night in, or while lounging in the bathtub with a glass of wine—and speak from a place of calm, factual clarity. This isn't about assigning blame; it's about fostering trust and caring for each other's health. Your diagnosis is just another chapter in your sexual story—one that doesn't define your desirability or your future.

THREE SEXY, SMART WAYS TO NAVIGATE HPV

Normalize the Conversation. If you've had HPV in the past, mention it as casually as you would any other common health experience: "Oh yeah, I had HPV once—super normal, and my body cleared it." HPV often lies dormant, meaning many people don't even realize they've had it. Since most of the population has been exposed, chances are, your partner has too. And if they react with shock? Educate them. Knowledge is sexy.

1. **Prioritize Your Health Like the Goddess You Are.** Schedule regular check-ups, get pap smears, and if you haven't gotten the HPV vaccine yet, talk to your doctor. If you smoke or vape, consider cutting back—it weakens your immune system's ability to fight off the virus. And yes, tell

your dentist to check for HPV lesions in your mouth and tongue—because oral cancers linked to HPV are on the rise. Advocating for your health is a power move.

2. **Reframe the Narrative.** HPV isn't a punishment; it's just another part of being human. Instead of seeing it as a blemish, think of it as proof that you've lived, loved, and experienced life. Confidence comes from knowing that your worth isn't defined by a virus—it's defined by the way you own your story, care for yourself, and move through the world with bold, unshakable grace.

3. **Pro-tip:** Ask your dentist to check for HPV lesions in your mouth and tongue—I've seen women as young as their twenties develop tongue cancer. Not to scare you, but to empower you. Knowledge is power, and prevention is sexy.

THE FINAL WORD: HPV DOESN'T GET TO WRITE YOUR STORY—YOU DO

HPV might be an uninvited guest, but it doesn't get to call the shots. The key to reclaiming your power? Stay informed, communicate openly, and prioritize your health like the queen you are. Whether you're nurturing a long-term love, embarking on a new romance, or celebrating your solo journey, remember: your sexual health is just one chapter in your epic, badass life story.

Stay informed, stay empowered, and above all, keep it sexy, honest, and entirely yours.

LESSON EIGHTY-THREE

SYPHILIS IS BACK—AND IT BROUGHT ITS MEDIEVAL MISCHIEF

WELCOME to the bedroom history lesson you never knew you needed. Syphilis—yes, the medieval mischief-maker of the sexual health world—is back. And like a toxic ex, it just won't stay gone. Let's get cozy, laugh a little, and learn why this ancient STD has made a twenty-first-century comeback.

THE GREAT IMITATOR: A DISEASE WITH A DRAMA QUEEN COMPLEX

Syphilis, caused by the corkscrew-shaped bacterium *Treponema pallidum*, has been called many things: The French Disease (by the Italians), The Italian Disease (by the French), The Great Pox, and the Black Lion. In Renaissance Europe, it was the OG STD villain. Shakespeare name-dropped it, syphilitic sores hid under those chic courtly "beauty marks," and famous figures like Oscar Wilde and Al Capone succumbed to its charms (read: they died).

But syphilis isn't just a dusty relic from history's naughty archives. In the past decade, cases have surged by over 250 percent. Yes, in the age of dating apps and sex-positive podcasts, syphilis is swiping right.

SYPHILIS 101: THREE ACTS OF TROUBLE

1. **Primary Stage: The Silent Intruder.** It starts with a painless sore (a *chancre, which sounds pretty but it ain't*) that might go unnoticed in the butt crack or the back of the throat. No pain, no shame, but contagious all the same.
2. **Secondary Stage: The Rash That Ghosts You.** Next comes a rash—sometimes on your palms, soles, or torso—that disappears without a goodbye. Unusual mucous patches can appear, too. Spirochetes don't send postcards.
3. **Tertiary Stage: The Mind-Bender.** Left untreated, syphilis can attack your heart, brain, and nerves, potentially causing dementia, paralysis, or aneurysms. It's not just a plot twist for Victorian poets; it's a real risk today.

WHY IS SYPHILIS BACK?

- **Complacency Post-HIV Crisis:** Modern treatments for HIV made unprotected sex less scary.
- **More Travel, More Trysts:** Love knows no borders; neither do STIs.
- **The Midlife Sexual Renaissance:** Viagra, hormone therapy, and newfound sexual freedom mean older adults are getting busy! (Yes, your parents might need a sex-ed refresher.)

SEXY, SAFE, AND SAVVY: TIPS FOR EVERY STAGE OF YOUR SEXUAL JOURNEY

1. **Get Tested Regularly.** Make syphilis screening part of your routine. "Honey, let's get checked together" is the new *date night*.
2. **Condoms Are Classic, But Not Foolproof.** Latex and polyurethane condoms help, though not perfectly. Syphilis loves a loophole—literally.
3. **Ask, Don't Assume.** A sultry whisper of *"When was your last STI test?"* beats an awkward trip to the clinic later.
4. **Watch for Mystery Rashes.** If your lover's got unexplained skin spots, channel your inner Sherlock. (Elementary, my dear vulva.)
5. **Own Your Health Like a Boss.** Swipe with intention, disclose with confidence, and treat knowledge as your best wingman (or wingwoman).

THE GOOD NEWS: IT'S TREATABLE!

Penicillin still reigns supreme. One shot can cure early-stage syphilis; later stages need more intensive care. If you're allergic, alternatives exist. And don't worry—there's no STD so scary that a little knowledge and proactive care can't handle it.

FINAL WORD: KEEP THE PASSION, SKIP THE PLAGUE

Syphilis may be a trickster from the past, but it doesn't have to define your future. Embrace curiosity, prioritize communication, and remember: sexual freedom and safety make the best bedfellows.

Now, go forth and live sexily ever after—with both passion and penicillin in mind.

LESSON EIGHTY-FOUR

MY, MY, MYCOPLASMA—THE SCARY LITTLE STD NO ONE TOLD YOU ABOUT

Darling, let's dim the lights for a PSA that's more cautionary than coquettish. Meet *Mycoplasma genitalium* (MG)—a stealthy little microbe as common as chlamydia but far less famous. Ignoring it? Not sexy. Knowing about it? Utterly empowering.

THE SNEAKY SCOUNDREL: WHAT IS MYCOPLASMA?

MG has been quietly crashing the sexual health party since the 1980s, infecting about 2% of adults, regardless of anatomy. It's passed through sexual contact—no penetration required. Symptoms often ghost you, but when they do show up, they include:

- **For penis-owners:** Watery discharge, painful urination.
- **For vulva-owners:** Unusual discharge, pain during sex, bleeding between periods.

MG can also cause urethritis and pelvic inflammatory disease (PID), jeopardizing fertility, comfort, and overall vaginal health. And yet, almost no one is talking about it.

THE TESTING TROUBLE: WHY MG IS PLAYING HARD TO GET

MG is elusive—there's no FDA-approved routine test. The nucleic acid amplification test (NAAT) is your best bet, using urine or a vaginal swab. But MG grows slower than a bad date's conversation, making detection tricky.

TREATMENT TURMOIL: THE ANTIBIOTIC CHESS GAME

Forget penicillin—MG has no cell wall to target. Azithromycin is the first-line antibiotic, but antibiotic resistance is a growing party crasher. Enter moxifloxacin, the 'big gun.' No sex for three weeks post-treatment—yes, patience is a virtue. And yes, your partner should be treated at the same time.

THE THROUPLE TROUBLE: A LESSON IN TIMING

A delightful throuple—two women, one man—taught me a lesson in synchronization. Partner One came in with classic MG symptoms, and testing confirmed the culprit. But Partner Three was out of town, delaying treatment. The result? MG played hot potato between them. Only when all three were treated simultaneously did they break the cycle. When it comes to shared love, shared accountability is key.

FOR THE LOVERS, THE LIFERS, AND THE CURIOUS CATS

- **Long-Term Partners:** Talk testing together— trust thrives in transparency.
- **New Relationships:** Chemistry's hot, but curiosity's hotter. Discuss STI tests, including MG.

- **Solo Flyers:** Notice anything unusual? Get checked. Self-knowledge is the ultimate aphrodisiac.

THE TAKEAWAY: CURIOSITY IS YOUR BEST PROTECTION

MG may be mysterious, but ignorance isn't bliss—it's risky. Advocate for yourself. This isn't included in standard STI screenings, so if you have unexplained, ongoing symptoms, ask your doctor about MG testing. Because in midlife, curiosity, cell cultures, and courage are forever sexy.

LESSON EIGHTY-FIVE

WHEN SEX HURTS—AND WHY WE SHOULDN'T JUST 'PUSH THROUGH' IT

Let's get one thing straight, my love: sex is supposed to feel good. If it hurts, your body is sending you a memo—and ignoring it isn't an option. You wouldn't keep wearing stilettos that make your toes scream for mercy, so why on earth would you tolerate painful sex?

Here's the thing: pain during sex is incredibly common. Up to 75% of women will experience it at some point, and between 20-50% of menopausal women deal with persistent discomfort. But common doesn't mean normal.

Painful sex can sneak up on you for all kinds of reasons—hormonal shifts, childbirth injuries, pelvic floor dysfunction, or even that enthusiastic yet ill-advised attempt to recreate that scene from *9 ½ Weeks*. It can be physical, psychological, or—most often—a maddening mix of both. And once pain sets up shop, it doesn't just live in your body; it takes up space in your mind, turning intimacy into something to dread rather than desire.

THE THREE BIG BAD WOLVES OF PAINFUL SEX

1. **Vaginal Dryness.** Public enemy number one. Caused by menopause, postpartum shifts, certain medications, and even stress. A dry vagina isn't just uncomfortable; it can trigger irritation, microtears, and infections. (Lube is love, lube is life—more on that in a bit.)
2. **Vaginismus.** Your pelvic muscles slam the door shut like a haunted house in a horror film—except, unfortunately, this isn't special effects. This involuntary spasm can make penetration feel impossible and is often a learned response to pain or fear.
3. **Vulvodynia.** A burning, cutting pain localized to the vulva with no visible signs. Imagine feeling like your underwear is made of sandpaper for no apparent reason. It can be triggered by infections, hormonal changes, or even allergies to soaps, condoms, or lubricants.

Now that we've met the villains, let's talk about reclaiming your pleasure.

YOUR PATH BACK TO SENSUAL BLISS

- **Talk Before the Touch.** Open conversations about pain shift the experience from *What's wrong with me?* to *How can I rediscover pleasure?* If you don't bring it up, nothing changes.
- **Redefine Intimacy.** Penetrative sex isn't the only way to connect. Explore sensual touch, erotic massage, oral pleasure, and other forms of intimacy that don't involve discomfort.

- **Experiment with Arousal First.** A well-prepped body is a happy body. Foreplay isn't optional—it's foundational. Clitoral stimulation, deep breathing, and sensual buildup increase natural lubrication and relax vaginal muscles.
- **Hydration, Lubrication, Celebration.** Moisturizing vaginal tissues with hyaluronic acid-based lubricants or estrogen creams can make a world of difference. And water-based or silicone lube? Non-negotiable.
- **Release the Tension.** Your pelvic floor holds onto stress like a bad ex. Kegels aren't always the answer—sometimes you need pelvic floor relaxation, yoga, or even a glass of wine before sex (yes, doctor's orders).

THE FINAL WORD

Your pleasure is not a luxury—it's your birthright. If sex hurts, something needs to change. Not your desire, not your worth, and certainly not your right to experience joy in your body.

So let's make a pact, shall we? No more suffering in silence. No more 'grin and bear it' sex. Instead, let's reclaim pleasure, one mindful, sexy, pain-free moment at a time.

And if you think this is the whole story? Oh, baby, we're just getting started. Up next: we go deeper—into the bedroom, beyond the pelvis, and straight to the heart of what makes deep dyspareunia a whole different beast.

LESSON EIGHTY-SIX

WHEN SEX HURTS, PART TWO—DECODING THE CUL-DE-SAC CONUNDRUM

We're talking about pain and pleasure—because one should never come at the cost of the other.

In previous lessons, we explored the front porch, the landscaping, and just inside the foyer (yep, the various parts of your lady house). Today, we're moving deeper into your palace—and perhaps into the backyard—to understand the mechanics of deep penetration pain, or what we in the medical field call deep dyspareunia.

THE CUL-DE-SAC AND WHY IT MIGHT BE GIVING YOU TROUBLE

Imagine your pelvis as a tightly packed grocery bag—full of necessities but crammed in without perfect symmetry. That's your uterus, bladder, rectum, some large intestine, ovaries, and all their connecting tissues. When something in that delicate ecosystem isn't happy, deep penetration can feel more like a battering ram than an embrace.

So what could be causing this discomfort?

THE HIDDEN CULPRITS BEHIND DEEP PENETRATION PAIN

Structural Issues—It's Not Just About the Vagina

- Fibroids or adenomyosis – Think of them as intrusive houseguests setting up camp in your uterine walls.
- Endometriosis – When uterine tissue migrates and causes sticky adhesions—like cobwebs turned to cement.
- Uterine prolapse – Gravity takes its toll, and things shift downward in unexpected ways.

Cysts, Scars, and Spasms—Ovarian Zits and More

- Ovarian cysts – Because sometimes your ovary decides to play hormonal roulette and grows a temporary, fluid-filled nuisance (exactly like a monstrous pimple).
- Pelvic adhesions – Silent, unseen webs of scar tissue making everything a bit too snug.
- Pelvic floor dysfunction – Tense, overworked muscles behaving more like an overtrained sprinter than the supple support system they should be.

Bladder and Bowel Blues—The Unsung Villains

- Interstitial cystitis – Bladder inflammation that makes any friction feel like a firestorm.
- Crohn's disease or irritable bowel syndrome (IBS) – Because gut distress often extends beyond digestion.
- Hemorrhoids – Yes, they can make penetrative sex an unexpected minefield.

WHAT CAN YOU DO? (BESIDES SIGH IN FRUSTRATION)

Painful sex doesn't mean the end of intimacy—it means getting creative with care, conversation, and solutions. Here's what I prescribe:

1. **Position Power.** Try positions where you control the depth and angle—cowgirl, side-lying, or even elevated hips with pillows can help you adjust the angle of entry.
2. **Slow and Sensual.** Deep penetration doesn't have to be the main event. Gradual, controlled movements and extensive foreplay can work wonders. Or play a game of "just the tip"—your body will let you know when it's ready for more.
3. **Lube Is Love.** Silicone-based lubricants last longer and reduce friction, making deeper thrusts more comfortable.
4. **Check the Angle.** Some bodies don't like certain positions. Experiment with pillows and slight shifts to find what works best. Side-lying positions can help prevent thrusts that feel like they're headed for your lungs.
5. **Pelvic Floor Relaxation.** Yoga, deep breathing, and even self-massage with dilators can help relieve tightness. And no, Kegels are not always the answer—sometimes you need to *relax* those muscles, not tighten them.
6. **Medical Check-In.** If pain persists, see a specialist. You deserve pleasure, not just perseverance.

THE BOTTOM LINE

Sex should be about connection and pleasure, not clenching your teeth and bracing for a swift kick to the lady taco. If deep penetration pain is your reality, know this: you are not alone, you are not broken, and solutions exist. Let's find the right one for you, so you can keep living—and loving—sexily ever after.

LESSON EIGHTY-SEVEN

MARATHONS, QUICKIES, AND EVERYTHING IN BETWEEN—HOW LONG SHOULD SEX TAKE?

HEY HEY, gorgeous. Banish the stopwatch and scorch the word *should*—sex isn't a race; it's a celebration of pleasure. Longer isn't always better, and faster isn't always worse. So, how long *should* sex last? The answer: as long as it's delicious.

THE RESEARCH RUNDOWN (AND ITS BLIND SPOTS)

- **1–2 minutes:** The sizzling quickie—short, sweet, and spontaneous.
- **7–13 minutes:** The *Goldilocks zone*, according to some therapists.
- **10–30 minutes:** The slow-burn session—perfect if you're savoring every second.

But here's the problem: these studies rarely count the laughter, the teasing, or the whispered *don't stop* that make it all unforgettable. While science is unabashedly sexy, most research times sex from *penetration to ejaculation*—heteronormative, clinical, and uninspired. What about pleasure before, during, and beyond? And hey, what about *us* gals?

CREATIVE PRESCRIPTIONS FOR PLEASURE

Play the Slow Game. You don't have to be horizontal to start foreplay. Send flirty voice notes all day, then turn your evening into a three-act play: a sensual appetizer (eye contact, soft kisses), a rich main course (full-body exploration without rushing), and a sweet, spontaneous dessert (a quickie tomorrow morning—no alarms needed).

Explore with Curiosity. Set a timer—not for performance, but for pleasure. Ten minutes of kissing only. Five minutes of hands-only exploration. It can even be a fun game: one person sets the timer, the other picks the activity. Then debrief in your briefs—what made your pulse race?

Indulge in Sensory Play. Light candles, grab your favorite toy, and play your sexiest playlist. Try edging—bring yourself close to orgasm, then back off. Build the tension and savor the release. Journal your desires for future rendezvous— with yourself or someone else.

THE BOTTOM LINE

Pleasure sets the pace. The best timing is *your* timing— whether two minutes or two hours. Forget the clock. Feel your body. That's the only *should* that matters.

LESSON EIGHTY-EIGHT

FREQUENCY AND FULFILLMENT—DEFINING YOUR OWN SEXY RHYTHM

Let's tackle one of the most persistent *shoulds* in our sex lives: *How often should you have sex?* Now, toss that outdated rulebook out the window, because the truth is, there's no one-size-fits-all answer. Whether you're having a sultry session once a month or lighting up the night daily, what matters most is that your intimate life feels fulfilling to you.

RETHINKING THE NUMBERS

We're bombarded with statistics: couples having sex once a week, twice a week, even twelve times a week—but remember, comparison is the death of joy (and a serious lady boner-killer). Studies show that couples who share intimacy at least once a week tend to be happier, yet that baseline is only meaningful if it aligns with your own desires.

Your *normal* is unique and ever-changing. Life is full of ebbs and flows—parenthood, work stress, or a shift in mood can all alter your sexual rhythm. Ultimately, satisfaction is the true metric, not the number on the calendar.

THE ART OF PERSONAL RHYTHM

Your sex life is like a well-tended garden: it blooms when nurtured in a way that suits your own soil. Instead of chasing someone else's frequency, tune into your body and your relationship. Ask yourself:

- *Am I satisfied?*
- *Does the quality of my intimacy fulfill me?*
- *Have I fallen into the trap of sexual inertia?*

Because when it comes to sexual well-being, *more* is not always *better*—what matters is that you feel connected, alive, and truly in tune with your desires.

SEXY STRATEGIES FOR SETTING YOUR OWN PACE

- **Craft Your Own Intimacy Calendar.** Instead of comparing your frequency to a statistic, create a shared *intimacy diary.* Note not only the times you're together but also the quality of your connection. Use these moments to celebrate growth, even if they're sporadic—it's all about evolving together.
- **Explore New Dimensions of Connection.** Expand your definition of sex. Incorporate playful experiments like a *sensual surprise* night where you explore nontraditional forms of intimacy: dancing, cooking together, or even tackling an escape room. Redefining connection can reinvigorate your relationship without the pressure of a strict routine.
- **Check in with Your Desires.** Set aside regular, judgment-free conversations about what you need. Ask, *What's my sexy state of the union?* This isn't about tallying numbers—it's about ensuring that you feel seen, desired, and creatively engaged. And if the

rhythm is really off, revisit *Lesson Sixteen: How to Stop Letting Mismatched Libido Affect Your Relationship.*

- **Start with Open Curiosity.** If you're in a new relationship, explore what feels natural without pressure. Share that you're still discovering your rhythm. This playful curiosity invites experimentation and deepens trust as you both learn what works for you.
- **Create 'No-Agenda' Dates.** Rather than considering sex as the final item on your to-do list, schedule couplings that prioritize spontaneity. Midnight walks, impromptu tapas at a cozy bar, or slow dancing in the kitchen—let intimacy unfold organically. It doesn't always have to end with something *in* a vagina.
- **Redefine Your Sexy Metrics.** Instead of asking, *How often do I get busy?* ask, *How pleasured do I feel?* Embrace quality over quantity. Reframing your self-assessment in terms of satisfaction rather than frequency empowers you to define what truly makes you feel vibrant.

THE TAKEAWAY

At the end of the day, studies have got it wrong: there's no universal blueprint for sexual frequency. Your ideal rhythm is as individual as you are—shaped by your desires, life's transitions, and the unique connection you share with your partner (or yourself).

If every song had the same beat and tempo, how mundane would music be?

What truly matters is that your intimate life nourishes you. Toss aside the *shoulds* and embrace what feels right.

Because your desire isn't a performance metric, a quota, or a competition—it's a rhythm that is uniquely yours. Trust it, honor it, and let it lead you exactly where you need to go.

LESSON EIGHTY-NINE

EAR-GASMS: THE PLEASURE OF LISTENING TO AUDIO EROTICA

Hey, hey, my sultry sound seekers—let's talk about the sexiest thing you can do with your ears. No, not that (well… maybe that, too). I'm talking about listening.

Think about it—podcasts are booming, bedtime stories for grown-ups are a thing, and audiobooks are selling like hotcakes. Why? Because listening allows us to imagine, to build a world in our minds that's uniquely ours. And now, my darling, we're bringing those listening skills into the bedroom. Or the bubble bath. Or the morning commute (no judgment, ever). Welcome to the world of audio erotica—sexy stories spoken straight into your ear, no visuals required.

FROM PORN TO PLEASURE STORIES

For years, video porn has been the go-to for a little, *ahem*, personal entertainment, but let's be honest:

- The plots? Weak at best.
- The characters? More wooden than cheap furniture.
- The body diversity? Basically nonexistent.

It's the same tired script: kiss, blowjob, cunnilingus, penetration, then a grand finale that somehow always lands on the eyelashes. *Really?* And let's not even get started on the ethical concerns, the dopamine overload, and the way too many extreme close-ups. Some of us are here for the fantasy, not a gynecological exam.

If you've ever thought, *Ugh, none of this feels sexy to me,* welcome to the revolution. Audio erotica ditches the over-the-top visuals and lets your imagination set the scene. It's like a choose-your-own-adventure book—except this one is way more fun after dark.

WHY WOMEN ARE FLOCKING TO AUDIO EROTICA

Fun fact: women are leading the charge when it comes to audio erotica. It makes sense—our turn-ons are often more mental than visual. Studies show that women use *mental framing* (a fancy way of saying "hot daydreams") to get in the mood. Unlike traditional porn, which is designed for fast, intense arousal, audio erotica is slower, richer, and way more immersive. It's less like a shot of tequila and more like a smooth glass of wine—you savor it. You sink into it. You let your own desires shape the story.

And the best part? You get to control the fantasy. Want the heroine to be curvy, tattooed, and in her fifties? Done. Prefer the hero with an accent that melts your brain? Easy. Every time you listen, you create a new version of the story—no weird camera angles required.

THE SCIENCE OF SEXY LISTENING

Listening to erotica doesn't just turn you on—it actually activates different parts of your brain than watching porn. Researchers have found that engaging with audio stories enhances creativity, deepens emotional connection, and even relieves stress. It's like meditation… but sexier.

HOW TO TUNE IN: A FEW SEDUCTIVE SOUNDSCAPES

Whether you're spicing things up, navigating a new romance, or enjoying solo pleasure, there's a way to make audio erotica work for you.

- **Make It a Pregame Ritual.** Listen as foreplay, letting the story set the mood. Pick stories that match your fantasies or surprise yourself with something new.
- **Send a Spicy Voice Memo.** Think of it as your own personal erotic audiobook. Whether it's a breathy whisper or a detailed confession, hearing your own voice can be just as thrilling as someone else's.
- **Treat Yourself to a Sensory Escape.** Cozy up with earbuds, dim the lights, and let your imagination take over. Try different genres, voices, and scenarios to discover what truly speaks (or moans) to you.

THE BOTTOM LINE: FIND YOUR FANTASY

Listening to a sexy story is about more than just pleasure—it's about reclaiming your own desires. It's about turning off the outside noise and tuning into *you*. It's about setting the scene you want, not settling for someone else's fantasy.

So go ahead—find a story, hit play, and let yourself get lost in the sound of seduction.

LESSON NINETY

SEX FURNITURE 101—BECAUSE YOUR BACK DESERVES BETTER THAN THE HARDWOOD FLOOR

READY TO ELEVATE your bedroom game (literally)? Let's talk sex furniture—because while your couch can double as a loveseat, a few well-placed additions might just save your knees, your back, and your dignity (RIP to that one pillow that never recovered from your experimental lube phase).

But is it worth the money? What even *is* sex furniture? And can you just grab something from IKEA and call it a day? Buckle up, my love, because we're about to break down the world of sensual seating, pleasure platforms, and furniture that does a whole lot more than just look pretty.

WHAT COUNTS AS SEX FURNITURE?

Sex furniture is designed to make intimacy easier, comfier, and way more fun—whether that means better angles, more support, or less awkward fumbling. Some pieces are discreet (looking at you, velvet chaise that doubles as a stylish lounge chair), while others scream *Wild Orchid: Home Edition.*

But not everything is fair game—wicker chairs, glass tables, and flimsy ottomans? Unless you have excellent health insurance, *hard pass.*

TYPES OF SEX FURNITURE & WHAT THEY COST

The Entry-Level Classic: Sex Pillows ($50–$250)

Think of these as the gateway drug to sex furniture. Shaped like a wedge (or a gloriously oversized cheese block), these little wonders help with hip elevation, back support, and better access for oral or penetrative positions. They can also be lifesavers if you and your partner have a significant height difference.

What to Look For:

- Firm but comfy (think memory foam, but sassier)
- Washable covers (because *you know why*)
- Portable and easy to store

Pro tip: Some of the most popular sex pillows? Originally marketed as children's play cushions—but once the parents figured out the real use, they flew off the shelves.

The Aerial Acrobat: Sex Swings ($100–$500+)

Ever wanted to defy gravity? A sex swing lets one partner hang suspended while the other(s) get full access without bearing body weight. It's a dream for deeper penetration and adventurous positions—without needing to hit the gym first.

What to Consider:

- Ceiling-mounted swings = permanent & sturdy
- Door swings = less commitment, more convenience
- Weight limit matters! (Read the instructions unless you want a trip to the ER.)
- Yoga swings? *Totally* moonlight as sex swings.

Pro tip: If you buy a ceiling-mounted swing, please use proper hardware. If it can't hold a chandelier, it probably can't hold your gorgeous ass.

The Chic & Sneaky: Sex Chaises, Lounges, & Chairs ($300–$2,000+)

For those who want style and stamina, meet the sexy furniture you can actually leave out in the open. These pieces look like elegant lounge chairs, but their curvy shapes mimic the body's natural form, making positions smoother and support stronger.

What to Look For:

- Soft but firm (like the best life advice)
- Easy-to-clean fabric (velvet? Gorgeous. Leather? Hot but high-maintenance.)
- Ergonomic designs to support multiple positions

Pro tip: Some of these pieces are so gorgeous, they look like they belong in a *Bridgerton* set. But trust me, they do way more than just sit pretty.

The Hardcore Classic: Sex Benches & Spanking Benches ($500–$3,000)

If you're kink-curious or just want a little extra support, these bondage-friendly benches are the go-to. Great for massage, deep penetration, and restraint play, they're adjustable, comfortable, and designed to keep things in place.

What to Consider:

- Height & padding (your knees will thank you)
- Some come with built-in restraints for added fun
- Usually made of sturdy wood or metal (because splintered sex is *not* the goal)

Pro tip: If you're not ready to commit to a full BDSM setup, a massage table can work just as well (and no one will question it).

Bonus Round: Fun Add-Ons

- **Dildo-mounted yoga balls ($50–$150):** Because why not bounce your way to bliss?
- **Waterproof sex blankets ($30–$150):** Fuzzy, cozy, and saves your mattress.
- **Rocking & motion chairs ($200–$800):** Like a rocking horse for grown-ups, but way more fun.

WHAT TO LOOK FOR WHEN SHOPPING

1. Fabric Matters:

- Velvet & microfiber = luxurious & easy to clean
- Leather = sexy but a nightmare for body heat & cleanup
- PVC/vinyl = easy wipe-down, but watch for cheap materials that might… *stick*

2. Stability Is Key:

- If one wild thrust can send it flying, skip it
- Weight limits matter (especially with swings & benches)
- If it's inflatable, make sure it stays inflated

3. Function & Storage:

- Some items fold away discreetly
- Others? Well… you might have to own them proudly

FINAL THOUGHTS: IS SEX FURNITURE WORTH IT?

Yes, my love! A well-placed wedge, an ergonomic chaise, or a sturdy swing can transform your sex life from *meh* to *mind-blowing.* Plus, who doesn't love furniture that *works* for you?

So go forth, shop smart, and remember: a good piece of sex furniture will never complain about your wildest ideas.

LESSON NINETY-ONE

HIGH ON PLEASURE—THE SENSUAL SCIENCE OF CBD

It's time to talk CBD in the bedroom! With millions Googling it and countless people swearing by its magic to ease anxiety and boost pleasure, we have to ask: are we all using this now in the bedroom? Get ready to dive into this natural, non-intoxicating wonder and discover why it's quickly becoming the must-have secret for unforgettable intimacy.

THE BODY'S OWN MIX

Our bodies produce a neurotransmitter called endocannabinoids—the *bliss molecules* that help regulate sleep, appetite, pain, and pleasure. This endocannabinoid system (ECS) even has receptors in our reproductive organs, setting the stage for a smoother, more pleasurable experience down there.

Cannabinoids are the active compounds in cannabis, one of humanity's oldest cultivated plants. The two headline acts?

- **THC:** The component of marijuana that lifts your mood and turns the vibe up to eleven, a.k.a. *getting high*. THC legality is as twisty as a pretzel, darling —it's legal for recreational use in some states while others keep it under lock and key. Always check your local laws, because wearing an orange jumpsuit isn't sexy at all!

- **CBD:** The chill, non-intoxicating partner that eases anxiety and promotes overall well-being. CBD won't get you high or tank your drug test when you stick to quality, hemp-derived products with less than 0.3% THC. Just look for reputable quality, and you'll stay clear-headed and test-safe.

A STORIED PAST & MODERN MAKEOVER

Cannabis has been used everywhere from ancient China and Egypt to the Greek and Roman Empires as a medical remedy for everything from glaucoma to childbirth, chronic pain, and digestive *woes*. Today, it feels like CBD is everywhere—from lubes and massage oils to patches and oral sprays.

When it comes to CBD in the bedroom, it's still early days, but there are some interesting science-backed uses. CBD may help:

- Reduce performance anxiety and promote relaxation (*anxiolytic effects*).
- Improve lubrication and blood flow via the endocannabinoid system.
- Provide pain relief for conditions like endometriosis or vulvodynia, easing discomfort.
- Potentially enhance arousal and sensitivity by reducing stress and calming nerves.

The research is promising, but, as always, it's still emerging, so more studies are needed to solidify these effects! Who wants to sign up?

BEDROOM BENEFITS & BEST PRACTICES

- **Topicals & Lubes:** Apply directly to increase sensitivity and promote vasodilation—hello, enhanced arousal!
- **Patches & Sprays:** Provide controlled absorption, giving you a discreet boost before the main event.
- **Oral Edibles:** A tasty way to calm nerves and set a relaxed mood so you can focus on the moment.

START LOW, GO SLOW

Whether you're using it topically or with a patch, begin with a small dose and allow 30–60 minutes for absorption. And please—always patch test on your arm first, *not* on your uber-sensitive genitals!

LEGAL & PRACTICAL POINTERS

Know your local regulations, especially if you're in a profession with frequent drug testing. Opt for products with minimal THC to stay on the safe side.

THE PLEASURE PRESCRIPTION: HOW TO MAKE CBD WORK FOR YOU

Massage Magic: A CBD-infused oil transforms an ordinary back rub into a sensual experience. The relaxing effects can reduce tension while increasing sensitivity—talk about a win-win.

Pre-Game Calm: Feeling a little performance anxiety? A few drops of CBD oil under the tongue about 45 minutes before go-time may help ease nerves without dulling sensations.

Lube It Up: Some CBD lubes claim to boost blood flow and increase pleasure—just make sure they're body-safe and free from irritating additives.

FROM ANCIENT REMEDIES TO MODERN PLEASURE

Cannabinoids are proving to be a game-changer in sexual wellness. Whether you're easing tension, increasing pleasure, or just getting a little experimental, CBD offers a natural way to enhance intimacy. Embrace the science, savor the benefits, and let nature's own aphrodisiac guide your way to potentially unforgettable experiences.

Enjoy the high life, my darlings!

LESSON NINETY-TWO

CLOTHING OPTIONAL—PLAN YOUR INNER SEXY SEX VACATION

IMAGINE your vacation not as a mere escape from routine, but as a *sensuous expedition*—a deliberate invitation to rediscover and celebrate your inner desire. In our youth, vacations often promised impromptu romance, salty kisses, and suntan oil that smelled like coconuts. But as we mature, the excitement of a *sexy vacation* can slip into a predictable routine—recycling the same beach clichés and tired resort packages.

But here's the delicious secret: you don't have to settle for the ordinary. Whether you're indulging in long-awaited solo time, rekindling passion with a partner, or simply redefining your relationship with pleasure, you can create an erotic getaway as spontaneous and vibrant as your own desires.

RECLAIMING THE ART OF EROTIC ESCAPES

The Mindset Shift. A truly sexy vacation begins in your mind. Before you even pack your bags, ask yourself: *What setting ignites my deepest fire?* Maybe it's a villa tucked away in Tuscany, where every cobblestone street holds the promise of a hidden rendezvous. Or a boutique hotel in Tokyo, where neon nights whisper secret adventures. Perhaps it's as simple as booking a charming hideaway in your own city, seeing it through fresh, seductive eyes.

Break Free from Vacation Inertia. It's tempting to stick to familiar vacation routines—hotel pools, poolside cocktails, and the predictable *dinner-with-a-view.* Instead, dare to experiment! Imagine a sunrise yoga session followed by a dip in a hidden waterfall pool, or a midnight skinny-dip in a private hot tub under the stars. Or a hot dude ranch where you can live out your Yellowstone fantasy (Save a Horse, Ride a Cowboy) Think beyond clichés—mix a little adventure with the spice of spontaneity.

Curate Your Sensual Environment. Think of packing as part of the foreplay—every detail should feel intentional and indulgent:

- **Revitalize Your Wardrobe:** Bring that silky camisole in a daring hue, the vintage little black dress reserved for *special occasions,* or sleek leather pants that make you feel invincible.
- **Set the Mood:** Tuck a travel candle into your bag (sandalwood, vanilla, or oud for that seductive warmth), a bottle of artisan massage oil, or a specially curated playlist that sends shivers down your spine—a *sexy mixtape.*
- **Design Your Sensual Bucket List:** Write down adventures like discovering a hidden speakeasy, booking a private gondola ride at dusk, or finally trying that new sex toy you've been curious about. Maybe a blindfolded massage or a daring role-play scenario is calling your name.

THREE SENSUAL TRAVEL ENHANCEMENTS

1. **The Sensual Story Swap.** Before your trip, write down a secret fantasy or a cherished memory

of an intimate moment. Maybe it's that sultry summer night in Santorini or an impromptu rendezvous in a Parisian alleyway. Then, during your getaway, exchange stories over candlelight and choose one to recreate—perhaps a midnight picnic on the beach, or a flirtatious meet-cute at the hotel bar where you pretend you're strangers.

2. **The Adventure Dare.** Embrace the thrill of discovery by planning one surprise activity that neither of you has tried before. Maybe it's a couples' cooking class where you create aphrodisiac dishes from scratch, a steamy tango lesson, or a scenic hike that ends in a secluded clearing perfect for whispered secrets and stolen kisses. The best intimacy often blooms from shared adventure.

3. **The Self-Love Sojourn.** If you're traveling solo, make your trip a pilgrimage of self-discovery. Enroll in a workshop on tantric practices or sensual meditation, book a day at a luxurious spa, or simply rent a cozy lakeside cabin where you can journal, paint, or explore pleasure on your own terms. Take a private dance class—imagine letting loose in a belly dancing session where every movement is a celebration of your own sensuality.

Pro-tip: Before you go, revisit *Great (S)Expectations (Lesson 17)* to keep vacation fantasies high and disappointment low. Because even the best-laid plans should leave room for spontaneous detours.

EMBRACE THE JOURNEY

Whether you're jetting off alone, with a lover, or curating an adventure in your own city, every sexy vacation is a chance to reinvent how you experience desire. Imagine yourself strolling along a moonlit boardwalk, indulging in an impromptu salsa lesson, or sharing a decadent candlelit dinner in a secluded chateau.

Every moment—from choosing an outfit that makes you feel *dangerously* attractive to diving into an unexpected adventure—can be a bold declaration of living sexily ever after. So pack that provocative lingerie, slip on your favorite heels (or bold sneakers, if that's your vibe), and set your inner compass to *seductive adventure.* Your next chapter of irresistible escapades awaits.

Now, go ahead—plan that sexy escape. The world is your playground, and pleasure is just a heartbeat away.

LESSON NINETY-THREE

HOT OR HOT FLASHES? HOW MENOPAUSE SPARKS SIZZLE IN OUR SEX LIVES

My darling, are you feeling hot, hot, HOT today? And I don't mean from the inferno of a hot flash—I mean the smoldering fire of pleasure and passion. Because here's the thing: menopause can absolutely ignite your sex life, not extinguish it.

THE MENOPAUSE MYTH: OUTDATED AND OUT OF TOUCH

Let's bust a myth right out of the gate: menopause doesn't mark the end of your sensual self—it marks your sexual renaissance. Forget the Hollywood script that says you're destined to become a side character in your own love story. It's time to rewrite that narrative. You're the lead, the femme fatale, the whole damn plot.

WELCOME TO YOUR SECOND ACT

Menopause is not a conclusion; it's a transition. Your ovaries have retired—moved to Florida, living their best RV life—but you? You're just getting started. Sure, there can be unwelcome guests like dryness, mood swings, and a libido that plays hard to get. But here's the truth: you are not your symptoms. You are the woman who will dance through them and emerge radiant.

THE SPICE AND THE SPITE: SEX AND MENOPAUSE'S DOUBLE EDGE

Let's get real about the tricky bits: hormonal shifts can be tricksters, lowering desire and making arousal more elusive. Your body may change, your moods may swing, and even your trusty clitoris might get a little shy. But remember, change isn't the enemy—it's the invitation.

THE UPSIDE OF THE 'PAUSE': PLEASURE WITHOUT PERMISSION SLIPS

Now, the pros—and they are delicious. No pregnancy worries, no monthly interruptions, just you and your desires front and center. Menopause is freedom. Freedom from old anxieties, freedom to explore, and freedom to say yes to what truly turns you on. No bleeding, no breeding—I always say!

PRESCRIPTIONS FOR PLEASURE: YOUR MIDLIFE SEXY BLUEPRINT

- Play, Don't Predict–Drop the ol' routine and get curious. What feels good now may surprise you. Explore with open hearts, hands, and a whole host of other items.
- Speak Your Desire–Honest conversations about your changing body can be deeply intimate. Expressing what sets you ablaze now is a power move.
- Lube is Love–Make it your bedside bestie. It's not a

crutch; it's a balm of bliss. Silicone, water-based—find your glide and ride.

- Own Your Radiance–Confidence is your sexiest outfit. Wear it like it's custom couture.
- Set Boundaries and Break Rules–Midlife is the time for clarity and playfulness. Communicate your desires and dare to explore.
- Slow Is Smokin'--Tease. Tempt. Take your time. Menopause invites you to savor every sensation.
- Date Yourself First–Invest in your pleasure. Self-discovery through touch, smell, and taste is empowering.
- Curate Your Fantasies–Books, toys, dreams—build a playground of desire for you, by you.
- Move That Gorgeous Body–Dance, stretch, feel alive. Erotic energy lives in motion.

YOUR MENOPAUSAL MIC DROP

Menopause isn't a cliff; it's a *launchpad*. This is where you stop asking for permission and start *owning* your pleasure. Now, just like all things in midlife, you gotta *warm up*. Whether it's erotic audio, ASMR, or something else, your foreplay needs are different at this stage of life. So, my loves, get out there and *live sexily ever after*. Because hot flashes may come and go, but *your heat?* That's *forever*.

LESSON NINETY-FOUR

LET'S GET PHYSICAL: HOW TO OVERCOME SEXUAL INERTIA

ISAAC NEWTON probably wasn't thinking about sex when he wrote about inertia, but let's be real—his principle applies *perfectly* to our intimate lives (bet you never thought you'd read Newton's name in a book about sex). Inertia, in physics, is the tendency of an object to remain at rest or continue in motion unless acted upon by an external force. In midlife, sexual inertia is that default state of *"not tonight, maybe tomorrow"*—until tomorrow becomes next week, next month, or... next year.

WHY DOES SEXUAL INERTIA HAPPEN?

Life. Gets. Busy. Work deadlines, caregiving, perimenopausal exhaustion, and those irresistible *just one more episode* Netflix nights creep in. Over time, your brain shifts from prioritizing pleasure to prioritizing, well, *everything else*. We tell ourselves, *"We'll get back to it when things calm down."* Spoiler: things NEVER calm down.

And here's the real kicker: the longer we go without prioritizing pleasure, the more our brain stops associating it with reward. Dopamine and oxytocin—the *get-you-hot-and-bothered* chemicals—drop, and the spark of curiosity dims. Before you know it, intimacy feels like another *task* instead of the juicy, pulse-racing pleasure it once was.

Sexual inertia isn't about lack of attraction or desire—it's simply the natural outcome of leaving pleasure on autopilot. But fear not! With a few tweaks, you can reboot your libido and get things back in motion.

FIVE PRESCRIPTIVE TIPS TO BUST THROUGH SEXUAL INERTIA

1. **Make Pleasure Appointments.** Yes, literally schedule it. Don't roll your eyes—if we can schedule Zoom calls and oil changes, why not *sex*? Routine primes the brain to *anticipate* pleasure, and anticipation itself builds arousal. Even if you don't feel *in the mood* right away, the simple act of *showing up* makes it more likely that pleasure will follow. Spontaneity is *overrated*—planning for intimacy is just foreplay in disguise.

2. **Change the Script.** If intimacy has become predictable (*same position, same bed, same order of operations*), shake it up. Try a new setting (candlelit floor picnic, anyone?), experiment with different kinds of touch, or shift the focus to non-goal-oriented pleasure. Sometimes, sexual inertia happens because sex starts feeling like a routine checklist. Turn it into a *choose-your-own-adventure* instead.

3. Build Anticipation Throughout the Day. Flirty texts, stolen kisses, a shared dirty joke—desire isn't a light switch; it's a slow burn. Keep the ember alive by weaving small moments of intimacy into your daily life. Your brain *loves* a good tease, and that simmering undercurrent of attraction makes it easier to flip the switch when the moment arrives.

4. **Prioritize Sensory Indulgence.** Touch silk, taste dark chocolate, listen to music that makes you *feel* something. Our desire is deeply connected to our senses, and sometimes reigniting pleasure starts *outside* the bedroom. If your body is in a rut, give it new textures, scents, and experiences to wake it up.

5. **Move Your Body, Move Your Mind.** Newton was onto something—motion creates momentum. Sexual energy thrives when the body is engaged. This doesn't mean running a marathon (unless that's your thing). It can be as simple as stretching in a way that feels delicious, dancing around your living room, or even just *breathing deeply* to reconnect with your body. Your libido isn't just in your mind—it lives in your muscles, your breath, and your movement.

THE MOMENTUM EFFECT

Inertia is real, but it's not permanent. The secret? *Start small.* One kiss. One touch. One moment of presence. Passion isn't lost—it's just waiting for a nudge. And like Newton said, *a body in motion stays in motion.* So go ahead—slip into the silk, light the candle, and give yourself permission to *feel.* Because once you do? Pleasure has a way of picking up speed. Now go, get physical—and let momentum do the rest.

LESSON NINETY-FIVE

THE SELF-CARE SCAM: WHY BUBBLE BATHS WON'T (ALWAYS) SAVE YOU

Let's be honest—self-care has officially jumped the shark.

What started as a gentle nudge for women to prioritize themselves has turned into yet another high-pressure, influencer-approved to-do list—one that's supposed to make us feel better but mostly just makes us feel like we're failing.

- Wake up at 5:00 a.m. and journal
- Drink a green smoothie
- Meditate for thirty minutes
- Take a bubble bath (with artisanal lavender oil, obviously)

The problem? Most women aren't doing these things—not because they don't care about themselves, but because they're busy, exhausted, and don't have time to turn their lives into a Pinterest board. Studies show that only 32 percent of women regularly engage in self-care—and I'd bet my favorite vibrator that most of them are just counting their morning coffee as 'me time.'

The truth? You don't need a self-care routine. You need self-love time.

WHY WOMEN SELF-SABOTAGE

Women are experts at putting themselves last. We sacrifice sleep, sanity, and sometimes our own health for our partners, kids, careers, and communities. We brag about how little we've eaten or how we "haven't sat down all day," as if exhaustion is some kind of achievement (who are these women who 'forget' to eat?? I have questions).

But here's the problem: burnout isn't a flex. It drains your inner sexy faster than a family holiday drains your energy. And let's be real—how sexy do you feel when you're running on fumes?

WHY 'SELF-CARE' IS BULLSH*T

Here's the deal: self-care should be personal. But instead, it's been repackaged into something generic, polished, and unrealistic—one-size-fits-all wellness. It's not that a bubble bath or a yoga class or binging *Mad Men* reruns can't be enjoyable for you. It's that those things aren't automatically the answer. Self-care, the way it's marketed to us, is another impossible standard; another way to feel like we're doing it wrong. Let's stop that now.

THE SELF-LOVE SHIFT: HOW TO ACTUALLY GIVE A DAMN ABOUT YOURSELF

Once women shift from the idea of self-care to self-love, it reframes the way our brains think about this time. Forget the spa days, the overpriced skincare routines, and the 'glowing goddess' affirmations (okay, we can do them some). Instead, ask yourself:

- What actually makes me feel good? (Not what *should* make me feel good, but what *actually* does.)
- What fills me up instead of draining me?

- What makes me feel sexy, powerful, and at home in my body?

Because when you truly practice self-respect, something magical happens:

- Your sex drive comes back from the dead (because pleasure is impossible when you're running on empty)
- You actually enjoy sex (because you're present in your body and not thinking about your inbox)
- You ask for what you want (because when you respect yourself, you stop settling—for bad sex, bad relationships, or bad anything)

THE TAKEAWAY: PLEASURE > OBLIGATION

Self-care isn't a list of things you force yourself to do.

It's whatever makes you feel like the best, sexiest, most alive version of YOU.

So if you've been waiting for permission to stop forcing yourself into someone else's version of 'wellness' and start actually enjoying yourself?

This is it.

LESSON NINETY-SIX

SEXY AT ANY SIZE: HOW TO STOP WAITING & START WANTING

Hey, hey, my luscious, luminous darling—let's talk about weight. Not in the *"should I eat the salad or the fries"* way (*fries, obviously*), but in the way it interferes with our sex lives before we even get naked.

How many times have you said (or thought):

- "If I could just lose 10 pounds, I'd feel sexier."
- "Ugh, I don't want them to see me naked right now."
- "Maybe next month, when I look better."

Sound familiar? It should—because almost every woman has felt this way. And I call **bullsh*t** on it.

The diet industry rakes in $71 billion a year, yet 95% of weight loss programs fail—meaning the only ones truly winning are the people cashing your check. And while the world keeps moving the goalposts on *ideal* bodies, we're putting our pleasure on hold until we look a certain way.

Well, screw that. Sexy isn't a number—it's a state of mind. And it's time we take it back.

SEX APPEAL THROUGH THE AGES: A REALITY CHECK

You know what was sexy throughout history?

- **Ancient Greece** – Big butts. Wide hips. Goddess status.
- **Medieval Times** – A round belly was *chef's kiss* perfection.
- **The Renaissance** – Women were celebrated for being soft, curvy, and powerful.

When did all this change? Oh, right—the late 1800s, when women were convinced to be weak, small, and delicate so they'd take up less space (*physically and metaphorically*). Then came the starvation diets, vibrating weight loss belts, and airbrushed magazine covers that convinced us that our worth was tied to our waistlines.

And yet, research shows our partners really don't care about our weight. Studies found that looking at a curvy woman activates the same pleasure centers in the male brain as alcohol or drugs. So while we're stressing over *those extra 20 or 30 pounds,* they're over there thinking, *Damn, she looks hot.*

So why do we keep holding ourselves hostage? Because we're taught to size up other women, compare, compete, and convince ourselves that we don't *deserve* pleasure unless we fit some impossible mold.

That ends right now.

HOW TO GET YOUR SEXY BACK AT ANY SIZE

Naked Time—Own It, Love It, Feel It. Spend five minutes every day naked—no mirrors, no judgment, just feeling your body (*vibing on her awesomeness*). The more you see yourself, the more normal and *desirable* your body becomes to **you.**

Turn the Lights ON. If you've been hiding under the covers, start slow—candlelight, dim lights, then full-on daylight sex. Remind yourself: Your body isn't the problem. Shame is.

Make It Historical. Have a toga night or recreate a Renaissance-style nude painting (à la *Titanic*). If you were a masterpiece in 1562, you still are now, baby—and worth a hell of a lot more!

Focus on Sensation, Not Size. Good sex isn't about how you look—it's about how you feel. Instead of overthinking, focus on the five senses to get out of your own head and into the moment.

Talk Sexy to Yourself. Would you tell a partner, *"Ugh, your stomach looks nasty in that position?"* No? Then why the hell would you say it to yourself? Flip the script. Compliment yourself—out loud.

Buy Sexy Lingerie for YOU. Not to *hide* or *fix* anything, but to celebrate your body exactly as it is. Get Pinterest-creative: a black lace bra and a white button-down shirt, a belly-dancing skirt with coins—dress to delight yourself.

Your New Mantra. *"I am not putting my pleasure on hold. I am not waiting to be a certain size to feel worthy, desirable, or sexy. My body is a living, breathing, pleasure-seeking force—and I intend to use it."*

THE (FAT) BOTTOM LINE

Sister, PLEASE stop postponing your sexiest, most confident self for a hypothetical future version of you.

The hottest thing about you? You—right now.

Go forth and be deliciously, unapologetically sexy.

Because even *the* Queen, Freddie Mercury, knew the importance of fat-bottomed girls.

LESSON NINETY-SEVEN

SEXUAL HICCUPS—LETTING GO OF GUILT & SHAME TO EMBRACE YOUR INNER SEXY

We're diving into those emotional hiccups that sometimes block our inner flame: guilt, shame, and regret. Think of this as clearing the air after a long, stormy night—making space for a fresh start. This isn't as flashy as discussing squirting or threesomes, but it's at the very heart of reclaiming our inner sexy.

Yes, we all stumble. Yes, we all have our moments of regret. And guess what? That's perfectly human.

UNDERSTANDING THE EMOTIONAL LANDSCAPE

Our sexual lives are not just physical—they're woven with emotions. Guilt, shame, and regret often join the party uninvited, making us question our choices, our desires, and sometimes even our self-worth. Whether it's feeling regret over a past misstep or wrestling with the weight of societal expectations, these emotions can dim the vibrant spark of our sexuality.

Imagine your inner sexy as a delicate flame. Every time you hold onto guilt or shame, you risk smothering that light. But here's the transformative truth: acknowledging and learning from these feelings is not a failure—it's an invitation to grow, to reconnect with the most authentic, passionate version of yourself.

THE ART OF MOVING FORWARD

Let's be clear: regret can be a wise teacher. It signals what we might want to change and empowers us to choose more nourishing, joyous experiences in the future. Instead of letting these emotions hold you hostage, we're going to learn how to set them down, make peace with them, and move forward with radical self-acceptance.

Here's your invitation: treat these emotional hiccups as stepping stones rather than stumbling blocks. They're clues—little whispers from your soul—guiding you toward a sexier, more liberated version of yourself.

HOW TO BUST THROUGH EMOTIONAL BLOCKS

1. Rewrite the Story in Your Head

Shame and guilt thrive in silence. Get them out of your head and onto paper. Write down what's haunting you, then reframe it as a lesson, not a life sentence. Example:

- **Shame Script:** *I made a bad decision that means I'm not worthy of a great sex life.*
- **Empowered Rewrite:** *I made a choice I wouldn't make again, but now I know myself better. My pleasure is still my birthright.*

2. Break Up with Sexual Perfectionism

Sex isn't a performance, and you're not being graded. Some encounters are magical, some are meh, and some are just plain awkward. If you've ever tripped while trying to strip or accidentally head-butted a lover (*we've all been there*), congratulations—you're human.

3. Unfollow the Shame Machine

If your Instagram feed makes you feel like you need to be airbrushed to deserve pleasure, it's time for a cleanse. Unfollow the accounts that feed your insecurities and start following those that celebrate pleasure in all bodies, ages, and identities.

4. Talk It Out—Even If It's Just to Yourself

A therapist, a trusted friend, even a voice memo to yourself—saying things out loud takes away their power. Name the guilt, name the shame, then remind yourself that you are not your past experiences—you are the person you choose to be now.

5. Build a Pleasure-First Ritual

When you reconnect with pleasure, you reconnect with power. Whether it's through touch, movement, music, or just wearing something that makes you feel like a damn queen, create moments that remind you that your body is not a battleground—it's a playground.

THE TAKEAWAY

Sexual slip-ups, missteps, and "oops" moments? They don't define you—they refine you. Think of them as detours on the road to radical self-acceptance, each one nudging you toward more honesty, more pleasure, and a whole lot more confidence.

When you own your story—stumbles and all—you turn guilt into growth, shame into swagger, and regret into a damn good lesson.

So here's your final assignment: forgive yourself, unbutton something (physically or metaphorically), and get back in the game. Whether it's a smoldering solo session, a toe-curling adventure, or just reclaiming the way you move through the world—own it, rock it, and for the love of all things holy, enjoy the hell out of it.

LESSON NINETY-EIGHT

THREE'S COMPANY: EVERYTHING YOU NEED TO KNOW ABOUT HAVING A THREESOME

Hey, hey, my ménage à trois-curious darlings—let's talk about the most popular sexual fantasy out there: threesomes.

That's right—95 percent of men and 87 percent of women have fantasized about adding a plus-one to their bedroom escapades. It's practically built into human nature. After all, some of the best things in life come in threes—The Sanderson Sisters, BLTs, Destiny's Child.

But while fantasizing about a threesome is one thing, actually doing it is a whole different ball game. It's sexy, sure, but it's also a logistical puzzle filled with rules, boundaries, and, ideally, fresh sheets.

So, whether you're just curious, actively plotting, or already making a hotel reservation, let's break it all down—the good, the steamy, and the oh, honey, let's not do that again.

IS EVERYONE REALLY DOING IT?

The stats are wild. Despite threesomes topping fantasy lists everywhere, only 24 percent of men and 8 percent of women admit to actually having had one. But let's be real—those numbers don't exactly add up, which means some folks either had repeat experiences or, let's face it, men might be exaggerating (shocking).

Meanwhile, dating and hookup apps report a 700 percent increase in people listing "threesome" as their top fantasy. And ethical non-monogamy? It's trending harder than espresso martinis.

Bottom line? People are curious. People are experimenting. And if you're one of them, you need to do it right.

Before You Jump Into Bed (Literally)

Here's Mama B's golden rules for threesomes:

- If your relationship has insecurities, a threesome will not fix them.
- If trust is shaky, a threesome will not rebuild it.
- If you're suggesting a threesome just to keep your partner happy… STOP RIGHT THERE.

Threesomes should be about shared excitement—not about "fixing" anything, not about obligation, and definitely not about jealousy-fueled chaos.

The Threesome Lingo You Should Know

- **FFM:** Two women, one man.
- **MMF:** Two men, one woman.
- **T in the mix?:** MFT or FMT, for threesomes inclusive of transgender partners.
- **Unicorns:** A bisexual woman sought by a straight couple for their ultimate fantasy (aka the rare, mystical third).

(And if you hear someone say they're "unicorn hunting," know that it's a thing—and unicorns don't like to be treated like sex toys.)

How to Bring It Up (Without a Panic Attack)

If you've been in a relationship for a while, saying, "Hey, what if we bring in a third?" can feel like dropping a bomb at dinner. So don't blurt it out mid-chew while your partner is working through a plate of chicken parm.

Start slow. Gauge their interest. Introduce it as a fantasy first and see how they react. And for the love of good sex—don't bring it up five minutes before the action starts. No one wants a surprise plus-one while they're already blindfolded.

Where Do You Find a Third?

If you're serious, dating and swinger apps can help. A few popular options:

- **Feeld:** For the ethically non-monogamous crowd.
- **Tinder:** Believe it or not, threesomes happen here.
- **Adult Friend Finder:** For the open-minded adventurers.

But whether you're a single looking to join in or a couple seeking a partner, remember: vet your people. Meet for coffee or drinks first. Set boundaries before anyone takes off their pants. And please—don't invite your best friend and expect things to stay normal afterward.

THREESOME ETIQUETTE: YES, IT'S A THING

- **Set clear expectations.** Who's touching whom? What's off-limits? Kissing—yay or nay? Establish ground rules before the action starts.
- **Use protection.** Unless you love awkward group STI conversations.
- **Keep the alcohol minimal.** One glass of wine? Sure. Enough tequila to forget your own name? Really bad idea.
- **Create an exit strategy.** Is your guest spending the night, or should an Uber be called? Plan ahead so no one feels weirdly stranded.

- **Check in afterward.** Whether you're in a couple or a single joining in, make sure you actually enjoyed the experience. No judgment, just honesty.

WHO'S THIS FOR?

Threesomes aren't for everyone, and that's okay. But if you're thinking about it, make sure you're going in for the right reasons: curiosity, excitement, and mutual pleasure—not pressure, obligation, or jealousy.

FINAL THOUGHTS: BEFORE YOU ADD A PLUS-ONE

Threesomes can be hot, thrilling, and even empowering—but only when everyone is on board, enthusiastic, and not just going along for the ride (pun fully intended).

If it's just a fantasy for you, enjoy it in your mind—it doesn't have to happen to be sexy. But if you do go for it, go in prepared, play safe, and most importantly—have fun.

Until next time, my love, as they taught us as kids, "Three. . . it's a magic number."

LESSON NINETY-NINE

SACRED SEXUALITY: WHERE THE DIVINE MEETS DESIRE

A<small>LRIGHT</small>, my love—let's get real about the kind of intimacy that isn't just skin-on-skin but *soul-on-soul*. We've covered the dirty, the playful, the uninhibited—but now, let's talk about the kind of sex that transcends. The kind that doesn't just make you moan—it makes you *wake up*.

Because here's the truth: sex has always been sacred. Not because some dusty old book said so, but because your body—your pleasure—was never meant to be anything less than holy.

But somewhere along the way, we forgot that. We let shame sneak in. We let rules and expectations dull the magic. We started seeing sex as something to hide, something to hurry through, something to perform—instead of what it was always meant to be.

A portal. A prayer. A power.

This Is Not About Religion. This Is About Reverence.

Sacred sexuality isn't about rules or rituals (unless you want it to be). It's not about lighting incense and chanting mantras (unless that's your vibe).

It's about seeing sex—whether with a partner, with yourself, or with the universe—as something more than just friction and release. It's about understanding that pleasure is not just physical—it's energetic.

It's a pulse that runs deeper than skin.

It's a force that shakes you from the inside out.

It's a moment where you are completely, unapologetically alive.

HOW SEX LOST ITS SOUL—AND HOW WE TAKE IT BACK

Once upon a time, sex was worship. Priestesses and goddesses were revered not just for their beauty, but for their connection to pleasure, to creation, to the universe itself.

Then came the shame. The control. The small, rigid boxes that told us what sex *should* be. Who it *should* be for. How much we *should* want it.

And suddenly, pleasure—our own birthright—became something we had to justify.

Enough.

Sacred sexuality is about taking it back. It's about rejecting the idea that sex is *just* about getting off. It's about slowing down, tuning in, and reclaiming intimacy—not just as an act, but as an art.

THE SACRED IS ALREADY IN YOU

You don't need a new partner, a fancy technique, or a tantra class in Bali to experience sacred sexuality. You don't need to wait for "the one" or for everything to be *perfect*.

Sacred sex isn't about who you're with—it's about how you show up.

WANT TO FEEL IT? TRY THIS:

1. Make Time for Seduction—Even If It's Just for You

Light a candle. Wear something that makes your skin feel electric. Breathe in deep and be in your own body. Desire starts with attention.

2. Let Pleasure Take Its Time

No rushing. No racing to the finish line. Slow. It. Down. Let every touch, every kiss, every breath be its *own* moment—not just a means to an end.

3. Bring Intention Into the Bedroom

Set a mood. A mindset. An energy. Whether you're alone or with a partner, let the space feel like a place of worship—where the thing being worshipped is you.

4. Breathe. Deeper Than You Think You Need To.

Breath fuels pleasure. It amplifies sensation. It keeps you present. Play with it. Drag it out. Let it take you somewhere new.

5. Feel It Everywhere

Sacred sex isn't just about *what's between your legs*—it's about what's between your ears, in your chest, humming in your fingertips. Feel it everywhere.

YOU DON'T NEED PERMISSION FOR THIS

Sacred sexuality is not something you *achieve*—it's something you *remember*.

You were always this powerful.

You were always meant to experience pleasure in its fullest, deepest, most breathtaking form.

So stop waiting. Stop apologizing. Stop *minimizing*.

It's time to step into sex that doesn't just satisfy.

It awakens.

LESSON ONE HUNDRED

HIEROS GAMOS: THE DIVINE, THE DIRTY, AND THE DELICIOUSLY YOU

Let's get one thing straight, my love: you were never just here for the sex.

Sure, we've explored the ins, the outs, and the oh-my-gods of pleasure. We've talked about vulvas, vibrators, and why angles matter. But beyond the mechanics, beyond the heat, beyond the breathless moans and the late-night fantasies—this entire journey has been leading you to one thing.

Sacred union. Hieros Gamos. The sexiest concept you've probably never heard of.

This is it, the ultimate Quickie—except, paradoxically, it's anything but quick. Because this, my love, is forever.

THE SUPER SACRED SEX YOU'VE BEEN MISSING

So, what the Helsinki is Hieros Gamos?

It's an ancient Greek term meaning sacred marriage, but not in the "let's register for a KitchenAid mixer" way. This isn't about a piece of paper, a white dress, or vows in front of Aunt Karen (thanks for the mixer, Aunt Karen).

This is the divine union of your masculine and feminine energies—the full embodiment of your most powerful, sensual, balanced self.

Hieros Gamos has been around for eons, whispered in mythology, carved into temple walls, acted out in sacred fertility rituals where priestesses and priests actually got it on to keep the crops growing (talk about job perks). It was cosmic, it was primal, it was sex in its highest form. And for centuries, women held the key.

Then came the repression, the shaming, the silencing. Sex became sin. Bodies became burdens. Desire became something to be controlled—until we forgot that sexual sovereignty was ever our birthright in the first place.

THE REAL SEX MAGIC—AND IT'S ALREADY IN YOU

Hieros Gamos isn't about a twin flame, a soul split in two, or the idea that you're only complete when you find *The One* (gag). You're not half of anything. You are already whole.

This is about the ultimate alchemy—where your divine masculine and divine feminine don't just coexist; they dance. Where you are both fire and water, both wild and wise, both warrior and goddess.

And when you truly embody this balance?

- **Your pleasure transforms.** It's no longer about chasing the next orgasm. It's about being fully present for every single pulse of desire.
- **Your relationships shift.** You stop looking for someone to complete you and start looking for someone who matches you. Who sees you, honors you, and—if you choose—ravishes you accordingly.
- **You step into your full sexual sovereignty.** No more apologizing. No more hiding. No more making yourself small so someone else can shine.

Because you, my love, are the whole damn flame.

SEX THAT TRANSCENDS THE PHYSICAL

Hieros Gamos is the ultimate energetic orgasm. This is sacred sexuality on steroids. It's where sex stops being just friction and starts being creation.

- Ever had sex so good you felt like you left your body? That's a taste of Hieros Gamos.
- Ever touched yourself and felt something deeper than pleasure—something like a homecoming? That's a glimpse of Hieros Gamos.
- Ever had a partner who saw you so completely, who made you feel so deeply, that your soul felt naked in the best possible way? That's Hieros Gamos in action.

It's not just about physical union. It's about the merging of body and spirit, shadow and light, surrender and power.

And let's be real—once you've had that kind of sex? You're never going back to basic.

THE ULTIMATE LOVE AFFAIR: YOU + YOU

Here's the truth: Hieros Gamos isn't something you wait for. It's something you step into. Today.

- It's the moment you stop chasing validation and start claiming your own worth.
- It's the decision to love yourself so deeply that you become untouchable in the best way.
- It's knowing that sex—good sex, soul-shaking sex —isn't just about pleasure. It's about power. Your power.

And when you fully, finally embrace that?

- **You don't just have better sex.**
- **You become sex.**
- **You become sovereign.**

YOUR INVITATION TO THE SACRED

So here we are, my love. The end of the book, the beginning of something much, much bigger.

You've had the power all along.

You were never missing a piece.

You were never incomplete.

You are whole.

You are divine.

You are the union of all things.

And when you finally feel that truth in your bones? Your pleasure, your power, your very presence will change the world.

Now go out there, and love, play, and claim your pleasure like a goddess.

Because you are one.

EPILOGUE

W‍HEW. You made it. One hundred little lessons later, and look at you—still standing, still fabulous, and maybe even a little sexier (if that's possible).

But here's the thing: this isn't the end. Oh no, darling. This is just the warm-up. Life didn't come with an expiration date on fun, pleasure, or confidence—and you've got decades left to flaunt it.

So go ahead—shake things up, say yes to the wild ideas, and remember: you're not aging, you're just getting dangerously awesome at being you.

Close this book, but don't close the door on your sexy, sassy self. Because midlife? It's just the beginning of your damn legend.

Now go out there and make 'em blush.

ACKNOWLEDGMENTS

To my freakin' fantastic kids, my partner, and my family—

Thank you for loving me through rants about the patriarchy, punchlines about lube, and my inexplicable need to talk about vaginas over cheese enchiladas. You are my reason and my ridiculousness. Kids: You can read this when you're 21. Honestly, maybe 41. But please . . . Someday read it.

To my writing circle at Gateless—

My fellow teachers, soul sisters, and word witches: thank you for bashing the inner critic one gorgeous, unapologetic sentence at a time. To the goddesses of Joshua Tree and the mystics of Southern France, the hive, the pod—I carry your magic in every draft. I'll never write alone again.

To the literary obsessives on Substack and beyond—

You make the internet bearable and brilliant. Thank you for reading, sharing, commenting, and showing up in my inbox with your beautiful minds and even better book recs. To my e-galley goddesses...divine blessings to you, sisters (Melanie Maure, Suzanne Kingsbury, Mariska Nicholson, August McLaughlin, Meghan Rabbitt, Jill Hamilton, and Kate Sukeforth.)

To my work in the world—

Menopause Rocks, the Institute for Women's Futures, Be. Women's Health & Wellness, and to every patient who has ever sat across from me and said, "Is this normal?"—

Thank you for trusting me.

Thank you for teaching me.

We need more education for women at midlife.

More education for all women.

Just. More.

To Alisa Kennedy Jones and Empress Editions–thank you for holding the vision and fighting for every line, every laugh, and every liberated voice. Even when the book was banned by the distributor as "porn." And thanks for sticking up for my cover, because as a wise writer (the Hive Pod) said to me, "No one— NO ONE—owns the pink zipper."

They were right.

We all have zippers.

And they are magnificent.

To my copy editor Valerie Costa, and to Kimberly Warner, David McLaughlin, Eleanor Anstruther, Ned Rust, David Roberts, Shannon Kennedy, Lisa-Marie Cabrelli, Kim Druker Stockwell, Alicia Dara, and the entire Empress crew—thank you for UNzipping the world with me. To Perfect Bound and Simon & Schuster, a hearty prayer-hands for rescuing us post-ban and giving this gyno a place to send her rebel wisdom to women worldwide.

And to my brilliant reader—

If this book made you laugh, sigh, clench, cry. . .

If it made you feel seen, or sexy, or just a little less alone. .
.

Then my work here is done.

P.S.

If you found this little note hiding here, then you're one of my people—the ones who read all the way to the credits, who cry at dedication pages, who check the copyright year and wonder what the author was going through.

Thank you for being the kind of curious, wild-hearted soul who knows the real magic is sometimes in the margins.

Now go tell your story.

And make it sexy.

Mulier. Libertas. Creatio.

(Woman. Freedom. Creation.)

P.P.S. I now understand the stress of an Oscars acceptance speech...what if I left out somebody??? To the wonderful somebodies I accidentally left out. . . I adore you.

ABOUT THE AUTHOR

Dr. Heather Bartos is an OB/GYN, menopause specialist, podcaster, author, and speaker, recognized as one of the nation's top five experts in menopause by Oprah Winfrey and Maria Shriver.

Her mission is to dismantle the taboos surrounding menopause and sexuality, empowering women through transformative midlife transitions. Leading the Menopause Rocks™ and Menopause Works™ programs, Dr. Bartos is at the forefront of revolutionizing care for menopause, both personally and in the workplace.

Her diverse background from PR to medicine to Reiki Practitioner and service in the Navy, underscores her holistic and personalized approach to healthcare. Featured in Shape, Glamour, Refinery29, ABC News, and named "resident gynecologist" by Poosh, her insights are pivotal in changing the narrative around aging and menopause. Cosmo magazine celebrates her as a 'supremely badass gyno,' highlighting her significant impact on women's health advocacy.

www.heatherbartosmd.com

If you have enjoyed this Empress Editions book why not telephone or write us for a free copy of the Empress Editions Catalogue and join us on Substack at TheEmpressAge.com. Our authors are also happy to join book club conversations. All Empress Editions books ordered directly from us cost $17.99 plus postage.

Empress Editions
303 Third Street
Cambridge, MA 02142

Telephone: +1 617.580.5266
hello@empresseditions.net
www.empresseditions.net